The Doctrine and Practice of Yoga

Including the Practices and Exercises of Concentration, both Objective and Subjective, and Active and Passive Mentation, an Elucidation of Maya, Guru Worship, and the Worship of the Terrible, also the Mystery of Will-Force

BY

SWAMI MUKERJI

YOGI OF THE SOUTH INDIA ORDER

1922

Republished from the public domain
by

Creative English Publishing

www.Creative-English-Institute.com

Under Classic Reads

August 2013

ISBN-13:
978-1492218494

ISBN-10:
1492218499

ANNOUNCEMENT

In studying these Lessons please remember 3 points:—

1. Not one useless or superfluous sentence is written. Every word is full of meaning. They are highly condensed. Think deeply over them.

2. They are meant as a practical supplement to the 'Spiritual Consciousness,' 'Soul-Force' and 'Inner Forces.' Studied side by side, these lessons will yield a great deal of benefit. You are expected to think hard and long.

3. Let none expect speedy or miraculous results. *All spiritual training calls for infinite patience and deep reverence unto the Guru. Constant rise and fall accompanies all progress.*

FOREWORD

Student! Your life is your own. You have only yourself to thank for what you are, have been and will be. Take your present into your own hand. Consciously shape out of it your future. Direct your forces along lines of study and endeavour that have the strongest attraction for you. Such attraction is the indication of need. It is the hand pointing out your Life-purpose. What your heart desires earnestly and clamors for incessantly is *attracted* to you out of the *invisible supply, i.e.,* the means, the environments, the right sort of persons, books and thought-forces are drawn to you and then you are expected to work out your desire. This is in perfect accord with the great *Law of Attraction.* Some call it God: since it answers all sincere prayers. Prayer, remember, is the sincere desire of the heart. I take it that you hunger for Truth and Spiritual Growth—else you and I would not be here. The instructions given you hereunder are meant to give you a strong body and a strong will. They will also tend to your Soul-Unfoldment. Talk not of them. Keep your mouth closed. Be serious, earnest and thoughtful. Then work at them confidently and with perseverance. Do not be daunted by apparent failures. Failure is the stepping-stone to Success. He fails who gives up a thing in final despair. Go on, I say. You will improve from the very first day, and in a short time you will be another man. All the leaders of humanity, past or present, have studied and investigated with tireless zeal along the special lines and, in Spiritual culture, you must do the same. But you must have health, a strong will and a steady brain, and I will enable you to have these positively. Keep these instructions strictly privately. Master them by constant meditation upon same.

Content

LESSON I

CONCENTRATION.

Concentration signifies the state of being at a center (*con* and *centrum*). Applied to thought, it is the act of bringing the mind to a single point. Each human being must practice concentration *subjectively* and *objectively*. In other words, each human being aims with more or less precision at concentration on a point *within* and a point *without* his own world. Concentration "without" is illustrated when you devote all your attention upon Nature, such as learning a trade, a profession, a science, an art or some form of business. This is *Evolution*, outgoing or positive mental energy. I shall call this; *Objective Concentration*. Concentration "within" implies the withdrawing of attention from the external world and the placing of mind on "God," "Spirit," "Heaven," "Religion," "Peace," "Nirvana," "Eternity," etc. This is *Involution, i.e.,* incoming or negative energy.

When *Objective Concentration* alone is practiced, you develop into a hard-headed, practical man of the world or a successful man of business. You are keen and shrewd. The world is a very matter-of-fact thing to you. You cannot think of anything else beyond money-making and pleasures and worldly affairs. You are a "worldling of the world," very clever, rich, and a master along your own lines. But spiritually you are an imbecile, worse than a baby. This is the *Objective Mind*—the "deepest immersed in matter, literally made of the dust." "It is the brain of worldly wisdom, common sense, prudence, methodical arrangement, order, discipline, classification, the skill and knowledge of the expert in any branch or department of art or science." This side of the mind is well developed in Scientists, Mathematicians and Businessmen, etc. Where it is not guided by the Subjective Mind, it can only see diversity and difference and is the slave of Maya—the slayer of the Real.

Subjective Concentration is seeking the Kingdom of Heaven *within* you. "God is Spirit and they that worship Him must worship in Spirit and Truth." LAPLACE, the great astronomer, asserted that he had swept the heavens with his telescope and found neither God nor Heaven. Yes, poor LAPLACE! He looked for God objectively instead of subjectively.

The Kingdom of God comes not with 'observation' but it is 'within' you. The be-all and the end-all of religion is the practice of Subjective Concentration. The performance of objective work by the human organism necessitates expenditure of energy and at last death, because all Objective Concentration means 'going from' the Absolute center—God— and hence it expends Spiritual Energy. Subjective Concentration means 'coming to' the center and hence it husbands and recuperates this energy. Now nature is motion to and from, and Spirit—the center of Life. This two-fold motion constitutes what is known as polarity—Evolution and Involution—negative and positive. At the negative pole life becomes involved, *i.e.*, 'wrapped up' in form. At the positive pole life 'evolves' or becomes expressed in nature. In Subjective Concentration you return for fresh supplies to the inexhaustible storehouse of force—the Absolute Will. Jesus healed the sick, exhibited control over external nature by raising the dead, because his chaste soul could receive nothing negatively from God and could give it out positively to the objective world. All power comes from God. I would impress upon you the all-important necessity of placing yourself in a magnetically passive attitude towards the Universal Will and then of taking up a calm, positive attitude towards the phenomenal world—which is a projection of the lower nature and hence must be handled masterfully, fearlessly and confidently. Be positive to the external world. Be negative and receptive to the Lord's Will-force. Remember this. This brings me to the supremest and most solid truth contained in the Science of prayer. The praying mind, by its mere attitude of faith and earnest expectation, opens itself out to the tremendous inflow of Divine Energy. It draws close to the center of all-power, wisdom and love, and drinks deep of the living waters of life so that even the very face or flesh begins to shine under the influence of this self-polarization—if I may be permitted to use this word—through prayer. Here is the *causa nuxus* between a prayer and its sure reply. Do you remember what Lord Rosebery said of the great Puritan Mystic Oliver Cromwell? If not, please let me quote: "The secret of his extraordinary success—he was a practical mystic—the most formidable and terrible of all combinations. The man who combines inspiration, apparently derived—in my judgment, really derived—from close communion with the Supernatural and the Celestial, a man who has that inspiration and adds to it the energy of a mighty man of action, such a man as that lives in communion on a *Sinai* of his own; and when he pleases to come down to this world below, seems armed with no less than the terrors and decrees of the Almighty Himself." Now both forms of concentration must be practiced so as to hold the two poles in the even balance of harmonious growth.

You will perform the daily work to which you are naturally adapted in the common weal (Objective Concentration) and after the daily task is finished, retire to the bosom of the Universal Spirit by the regular practice of Subjective Concentration.

Now will you realize the ideal of peace in the very midst of the toil and sweat of the day.

The foregoing diagram, if closely and thoughtfully studied, will show the stages the mind has to 'grow into' in objective and subjective concentration.

In order to acquire knowledge of the laws of external nature the mirror you require is accurate observation and you must focus your attention and push objective concentration to its final stage of perfect knowledge or illumination in order to master any special branch of science.

In Objective Concentration , Pratyahara and *Dharana* are the preparatory stages. Take a scientist, for instance. He knows that when the mind is engaged with several things, mind force is scattered. He cannot be a politician, a musician, etc., and at the same time an expert scientist. He gradually abstracts his attention from all other subjects and pauses it on one subject or one set of subjects.

Pratyahara is the continued effort of the mind to so abstract itself.

Dharana is reached when this effort is finally successful and the mind becomes steadfast and one-pointed. *Dhyana* is an extension of this steadfastness. When *Dhyana* is reached, the student is beyond the range of books. His mind is occupied with original researches and experiments and his knowledge becomes more and more definite. Going on and on always on the one line complete knowledge of that subject is attained. This is the objective view of *Samadhi*. All these stages when completed make one *Samayana*. The subjective view of *Samadhi* no books or writings can teach you. As you go deeper and deeper into Yoga, you will understand these things in the light of your Soul-Vision. It will come to you if you follow my subsequent instructions. Despair not.

WHAT IS MAYA?

Now, first of all, what is Maya (ignorance of the real)? Take the dial-plate of a watch. You know quite well that the hands of the watch are governed by the mechanism behind. Both are necessary. Ignorance exists in thinking that the hands of the watch move by themselves. This visible universe is the dial-plate of the Invisible. Maya (ignorance) blinds you to this fact, *i.e.*, mere objective knowledge blinds you to the subjective side of life and you see nothing beyond a material universe. But you, who realize both, objective as well as subjective, need not be afraid of such a danger. For a danger it is to develop the objective mind die neglect of the subjective. In order to round yourself out, practice both. *But first, last and always, let the subjective guide, govern and illumine the objective.* Also remember this: If your mind is at all attached to the objective world, try your very best to dis-attach it and fix it on the subjective side of life, else will you bring untold suffering on yourself. The half-wordly and half-spiritual man who wants to lead a spiritual sensual life eventually brings about a conflict between the laws and forces of the two planes of being. He is overwhelmed with pain and at last with cries of suffering, disease and loss, he is made to open his eyes. Understand the world for what it is but do not lower your soul to the point of being attached to its small thoughts, things and ways.

HOW TO CONCENTRATE OBJECTIVELY.

(*a*) In all undertakings whether of small or great importance shut off all thoughts and ideas except such as have any immediate and direct bearing upon the thing in hand. Pay attention. Bend all the energies of your mind and will upon it till it is completed to your satisfaction. Divert your attention from one thing to another only when you sanction by a resolve and understand why you do so. Your daily work which you must choose according to the special bent of your mind, will present you opportunities.

(*b*) Control impulse. Suppose an idea enters your mind. Compose yourself quietly before carrying out its purport. Consider it. Turn it over in your mind. Contemplate it. Weave your mental energies around it, as it were, till at last the idea with your final decision stands out clear-cut and well-defined. Then proceed to act it out physically with your mental concentration cutting a way for you straight on to the execution of your designing. This is *forethought*.

(*c*) In perfect concentration time vanishes. In working out a design on which you have set your heart dispense altogether with the element of time and work at it concentrated for days, months and years with confident expectation of success.

(*d*) Take a picture, representing a landscape, the interior of a building, an assembly of persons, a square, a triangle or a more complicated geometrical figure. Look at it well. Then lay it aside. Close your eyes. Reproduce the picture mentally in detail. Then repose your mind on the same image to the exclusion of all other thoughts. This is a more fixed and meditative method and will sharpen the mind wonderfully. It will also develop the power of conscious Mental Imagery. The key to Objective Concentration is *Conscious Attention*, remember.

ACTIVE AND PASSIVE MENTATION.

These terms imply two different distinct functions of the human mind. The active function performs the volitional, voluntary thinking. It is the conscious focusing of the mind on some mental problem. Banishing from the mind all thoughts and ideas not in harmony with your special subject of study implies Active Mentation. This function is used by the active, wide-awake man in his busy and energetic moments. It is the key to the development of Will-Power and a vigorous intellect. You are conscious of effort when you are exercising this function. The mind becomes exhausted after a great deal of such effort and cries out for rest, because conscious attention implies close concentration of thought and can be exercised only by the conscious use of Will-Power. You ought to be able to concentrate upon one subject of thought, study and observation with undivided attention and then take your mind off that subject and put it on something else, at your will. Train your mind to 'give' perfect attention to any subject you like and also to 'shut off' or inhibit all attention on that subject. The mind is a restless thing darting from one thing to another, and, like a spoilt child, tiring of continued attention. But you must, by Will-Exercise, get control over this tendency. 'Exercise develops power. Practice makes perfect.' This you must bear in mind and, by patience and perseverance, train your mind to 'pay attention' where it ought to do so and not to pay attention where it ought not to. At first your mind will rebel like an unbroken horse at the imposition of such restraint. But really all greatness results from mind-control. *Remember active mentation is conscious, deliberate concentration. Passive mentation represents automatic, involuntary thinking.* This includes the subconscious or 'habit' mind. When a certain thought-groove has been formed in your mind, energy flows into it involuntarily, *i.e.*, by itself and without any conscious effort on your part. This is passive mentation. It is automatic mental activity. Take an example. Some school-boys find Mathematics, Science and Geography easy to master from the very start. They feel quite in sympathy with the teacher of Mathematics. But History and Language are their abomination. There are others who simply cannot 'take an interest' in any Mathematics but who shine brilliantly in Language, Recitation, Composition, History. As a matter of fact neither of these students is superior to the other, but each is great in his own line. In one set, you have an example of automatic mentation in Mathematics, Science and Geography; in the other in Literature and Art. But suppose the first set tried to master Literature and Art and the second grappled with Mathematics and Science, each would then be practicing actual concentration. In each set the active function would be exercised and will-power would develop on both sides. Do you see? Occultists say that all power results from the continual exercise of active mentation and all weak-mindedness is the direct outcome of this wool-gathering, castle-building, inattentive habit which is an extension of passive mentation into useless channels of thought-force. Conscious attention concentrates and even specializes mental energy as the sun-glass concentrates and intensifies the heat of the rays of the sun. Focus your full attention upon the thing to be done, take a keen interest in its accomplishment to the exclusion of all else, and you will obtain wonderful results. The man of developed, concentrative power holds in his hand the key to success, with the results that all his actions, voluntary or involuntary, are pointed to the accomplishment of his object. Remember therefore in conclusion:

(1) Concentration is perfect attention consciously directed to a given point of achievement either objectively or subjectively.

(2) Concentration is consecration.

"Whatever you do, do it with all your might. Do one thing at a time and do it well." By concentration is meant the directing of all your energies along a special line of achievement. For instance, if you would be a perfect Yogi, you must concentrate, concentrate, morning, noon and night, at all times, along that line of endeavor. You must study all the vast literature on Yoga, Psychology, Metaphysics, Mentalism, etc., and form your own synthesis on same. You must think hard and work hard for Yoga. "Genius is the power to bear infinite pain." Nothing ought to be too great a sacrifice, including your own life, for the right understanding and achievement of Yoga.

All half-heartedness, all insincerity, weakens your nature, and weakness has no place either in heaven or in hell. For the half-hearted man is a traitor unto the Divine within him and must pay dearly for his treachery.

SUBJECTIVE CONCENTRATION — HOW PRACTICED.

This is a vast subject. If you practice earnestly my instructions on Thought-Control, Will-Culture, and take the Meditation Exercise I am going to give you, you will realize greater strength than average humanity. But you must study and think hard for yourself before any considerable benefit can be derived from even these. Remember please, you alone can teach yourself through intuition. Intuition is tuition from within. Follow strictly the general rules I give you and you cannot but unfold your Inner Soul Vision which includes intuition in its fullest sense.

(a) What is Thought-Force?

"Thoughts are things." Thought is a dynamic energy. Just as the food that you eat feeds your body, exactly similarly your thoughts and feelings nourish your soul. Matter is nothing but a concentration of Thought-Force or Mind-Substance. The entire universe is seen objectively. This is on the cosmic scale. On the individual scale—"As a man thinks in his heart, so he is." This is a literal truth. Your body is nothing but a Thought-Form. Control your modes of thinking and shape them to lofty ideals. So will you infallibly, positively and immediately control your destiny. Control your thoughts and you can control the thoughts of all other men. The tone of your thoughts must always be lofty.

You must change your Thought-Habits and shift your plane of consciousness from the lower to the higher life. I am going to give you hints on same. Pay attention please.

(b) Thought-Forms.

Every one of us, as he thinks, feels and wills, sends forth Thought-Forms and Thought-Waves of greater or lesser intensity. This force once set into motion persists, for a greater or lesser period of time, in Ether. Thought-Force is the concentration of a high form of vibratory energy in the Akasa (universal ether) and the ether, as you know, permeates all space, interpenetrates and pervades all forms of matter, from atom to the sun and the stars. Just as the light-waves of a star exist and move on centuries after the star has ceased to be, just as the heat-vibrations remain in a room even after the producing cause has been removed, similarly mentative energy and its corresponding Thought-Forms persist in the ether even after the originating impulse has been withdrawn.

(c) Thought-Atmosphere.

In this way places, houses, cities and temples have peculiar Thought-Atmospheres of their own, imparted by those living there, exerting an influence upon every one living or going there. These are positive, animating, purifying and exalting Thought-Atmospheres, and there are negative, weakening and unholy, morbid Thought-Atmospheres.

The higher and loftier your tone of general Thought-Activity, the finer and more powerful the vibrational nature of the energy emanating from you. The quality of the thought determines the rate of vibration. For instance, photographs have been taken through highly-sensitized plates, indicating the nature of the energy generated. Tongues of flame, brilliant and flashing with golden-yellow, were photographed from prayer and devotion. Rotary forms spreading out in ever widening circles of intense power appeared from lofty enthusiasm in a noble cause. Dark, murky, cloudy forms resulted from fear, morbidness and worry, and so on.

(d) The Human Aura.

Similarly each human organism has an 'Aura' of Thought-Force around it, having its own peculiar rate of vibration, its peculiar forms of color, etc. This 'Aura' is an extension of our physical, mental and spiritual energies.

(e) The Adductive Power of Thought.

Now as you think, the quality of your thoughts and feelings sets up a magnetic center within your Aura, vortices are created, attracting to yourself similar forms of thought and mentative energy and combining with other similar forms of energy, reacting upon you and your circumstances and also wielding an influence upon all such as may come within its area, radius or field of Force. Thus you see thoughts of the 'I can and I will', 'I do and I dare' type draw similar ones to you, ever increasing your own stock and at the same time stimulating and energizing all others vibrating in the same key throughout the world. Hence you see we owe it to ourselves as well as to humanity in general to generate only positive, loving and lofty thoughts. Just brace up and send forth fearless, 'I can and I will' thoughts into the world's great reservoir of thought forces, and you will be surprised at your power to attract influence, and energize others.

(f) Thought-Control.

There are four special classes of thoughts that are poisoning the lives of almost all humanity. They are:—(1) Fear-thoughts, (2) Hate-thoughts, (3) Sensual-thoughts, (4) Selfish-thoughts. All worry, doubt, timidity, lack of self-respect, jealousy, spite, malice, envy, slander, dirty, vicious, will-weakening, health-destroying, poverty-breeding, soul-killing influences radiate from one or all of these four. You must cut at their roots and utterly destroy them. In your efforts follow assiduously the following four rules. They alone can give you absolute thought-control. They are infallible:

(1) You can break up old thought-habits and build up new ones by sheer force of Will.

(2) You can easily become great by associating with some strong-willed, holy, wisdom-steeped soul. This is absolutely necessary and means the finding of your Guru.

(3) By auto-suggestion, *i.e.*, by impressing upon your passive mind the particular change you would have it work out.

(4) By thought-absorption, *i.e.*, by constant meditation on that one line of thinking.

Now let me give you a few valuable hints on the above four in detail:

(1) & (3). *Character Building*.

You can accomplish this result by tensing the will and by strengthening the active function of your mind and thus enabling it to "step in" and simply 'command' the passive function to drop the old thought-habit and take up the new one. This is a magnificent feat and in it only the strongest succeed. You can obtain good results by combining this with auto-suggestion. Silently concentrate upon your passive mind and impress upon it your order. Say to it earnestly, confidently, and masterfully: 'You, my mind, I want you to be fearless, pure, loving and unselfish!' Picture to yourself in imagination as if you were already these, and again command and impress your will upon your mind. Do so silently and constantly and never neglect a chance of expressing these qualities in action because, at first your mind will rebel, but if 'you' keep up your efforts determinately and firmly and avail yourself of all opportunities to 'act out' your will, your mind will end up by accepting your suggestion and manifesting same naturally as a habit. Some of you will actually go out of your way to 'act out' a thought when you realize that the easiest and surest way to check and utterly 'destroy' a thought-habit is to refuse deliberately to let it manifest in action and to 'create' a new one all you have got to do is to equally deliberately 'express' it in action and thus clinch it into permanent strength. Also you must aim at 'thoroughness' and guard against all compromise with your lower nature. Chastity must be perfect chastity and nothing short of that, and so on in all development.

(4) *Thought-Absorption.*

i. Go away by yourself to some place where you will not be disturbed. Of course, not always and very rarely can you obtain this condition. Never mind. Do your best where you are and the great law will at least find for you all necessary conditions. Shut out all distracting conditions and impressions from the outer world. After a little effort you will be able to do so anywhere, at any time, and under any condition. All mental disturbance is within you.

ii. Now relax, go passive, and draw off all tension from your nerves. Just you relax your mind and your body will follow suit. A few deep slow breaths will help the beginner.

iii. Concentrate upon your mind inward steadily, calmly and with undivided attention.

iv. Fix your thought firmly upon your passive mind and mentally say, 'You, my mind, are quite *pure*.' Think of this word (with all the ideas associated therewith) as sinking deeply into your mind and making a deep impress upon it as a die upon a wax. Let the outward form of the words 'pure,' 'fearless,' etc., sink into your mind.

v. Form a mental picture of yourself as if you already possessed all 'purity' and 'courage' and act them out in imagination. Make of it a pleasant 'day dream.'

vi. Intensify your relaxed condition of mind. Grow as 'limp' as a rag. Then mentally open yourself out to the inrush of all the Thought-Forces existing in the ether and connected with positive thoughts. The effort of this imagination to see this tremendous force pouring into your brain and body will actually put you *en rapport* with same.

vii. Now change from negative to a positive condition and say vigorously I am '*pure*' and '*strong*' Say it distinctly several times. Actually speak them out.

viii. Then go out and *live your thoughts out*. This last is the most important condition.

ix. Practice this daily at the same hour and if possible at the same place, morning and evening. In fact hold the thought in your mind as often as possible till it becomes second Nature.

x. Use your power for good or you shall weep eternally. To misuse occult powers for mean, selfish, or low ends and to prostitute it into enslaving others weaker than yourselves mentally and physically is the greatest 'sin' man can commit against man.

(2) *Guru Worship*.

You grow by absorption and assimilation. In order to quicken your progress you need abstract as well as concrete ideals. The secret of all rapid and startling spiritual development is man-worship. By man-worship I mean devotion to, reverence, and intense and all-absorbing passion for the perfect individual man of realization—a Mahapurusha. Christ, Buddha and Vivekananda were all such-type men. You must constantly and thoughtfully meditate upon the lives and writings of saints and heroes. The formative influence and valuable powers of study and meditation upon lofty ideas and ideals are incalculable. Man grows by the deepening of consciousness and the acquirement of wisdom. All study, subjective and objective, is a *Tapashya* or Austerity directed to the acquirement of wisdom. It is the worship of Saraswati—the Goddess of Wisdom. This worship is definable as perfect emotional solitude, close study, absolute chastity and celibacy, and at last the merging of the personal into the impersonal. This austere life is the secret of all greatness. You know how Archimedes when threatened with death by the vandalistic invaders of his country raised his head and said 'Please do not disturb my circles' and nothing more. This man was practicing Yoga unconsciously. You must be able to lose all consciousness of this relative personality, the sure victim of death and impermanence. You must give up the personal ego that in the words of Walt Whitman 'is contained within your hat and boots' and then alone will you realize an infinite individuality. Truly in losing himself man finds Himself. 'Ye must be born anew'. Herein, apart from its formative and moulding influence lies the greatest value of study. Study and direct aural influence of a perfected soul are the two objective means of instilling powerful suggestions into the subjective self or the inner soul. All knowledge is within the deeps of the eternal subjective. But the gate is locked. Your Guru gives you the master-key with which to unlock the door and enter the gate of wisdom and power. Once you are there all pain and death shall be conquered. You can then help yourself. Man can only worship such a God as is greater than himself in degree and not in kind. Such a God he can "grow into." It is the impersonal God of the Hindu Philosophy that gives you the abstract ideas and the living Guru (God) in human form that gives you the concrete ideal. The one is necessary for the soaring intellect; the other for the rousing and enkindling of tremendous and indomitable motive-power. Seek both and when you find them worship and serve them with all your heart and soul. 'My worship for my master is the worship of a dog. I do not seek to understand his nature. It ever startles with its newness and profound depth'. So spoke Vivekananda of Ram Krishna. Need I tell you of the tremendous and world-conquering power that awoke in Vivekananda through mere Guru worship? In India the Guru asks for nothing short of absolute worship, obedience, and submission to his will although none values and appreciates individual freedom more than the master. So long as you are at the feet of your master be as submissive as a lamb. So will you open yourself to his great batteries of inner power. Serve him. Please him. Obey him. Be his slave. No matter what contradictions you may see. A great and profound nature is full of contrary ways and his character is a paradox impossible for you to read through reason and observation. You can only understand him by having perfect faith in him, loving and serving him like a faithful dog. So will you tap on to his inner forces. And when he sends you away into the broad world to live out the great ideal he has set before you, you shall be astonished at your courage and power. You shall take fearless possession of this world and every minute you shall realize how only he can command who has learnt to obey. By commanding I do not mean dominating any one and forcing your views on others. This is the sign of fools. But you will find your influence radiating and circling out naturally and irresistibly, winning souls to the higher life, and you yourself shall thus stand as a tower of strength, a redeemer of the race, an inspiration and a living benediction unto humanity. Peace be with you! May you realize strength of soul!

LESSON II

PERSONAL MAGNETISM, WILL-CULTURE, SELF-CONTROL.

Personal Magnetism is the individual expression of a subtle irresistible and dynamic *Force* in man, which enables him to exert an unusual influence upon others. You all have come into contact with men of this type. They are endowed with marvelous, almost miraculous powers of influencing, persuading, attracting, fascinating, ruling and bending to their own Will-Force men of widely varying mental peculiarities and temperaments. Men actually go out of their way to please them. They attract others without any visible effort and others feel drawn to them in spite of themselves. Various are the examples of such power as afforded by history.

Now what is this power due to? How to develop it within yourself? Is it possible for everyone to acquire it? Has it or can it be put to any higher and nobler use than merely to enslave others' minds in order to make them subservient to your selfish purposes on the relative plane of existence? If so, what is that higher use? I know of a Christian gentleman, Mr. K. by name, who had been smitten with the young governess of a Magistrate in Benares. This grown-up man sought out a young College student who was a born leader of men and who was adored, admired and universally respected by all students, teachers and professors. "I wish you would teach me Mesmerism so that I may *fascinate* that girl"—this was the application of Mr. K. Well, the upshot of it all was that Mr. K. got a severe and stern rebuke from the young mesmerist, who in all truth was a born Yogi and cared not for the petty ways and small thoughts and attainments of men of this world. I find that nearly all modern Western writers on and teachers of this subject are much, in fact solely, taken up with the idea of sensationalism through Occultism, so much so that when a really thoughtful man investigates their writings he feels utterly disgusted, repelled and horrified at the very name of Occultism. "*It is sin to manifest power*," said Vivekananda. The man who studies Yoga and Occultism simply with a view to develop, display and demonstrate Psychic and Super-normal Powers and *Siddhies* always ends in *Lust* and is caught up in a psychic machinery of law and destructive thought forces that effectually grind him to pieces. His spiritual progress is thrown back over ages and he is made to retrace his steps slowly and painfully. I cannot too strongly condemn the modern tendency to "impress" others, to "strike terror" into others, to "psychologize" others towards the accomplishment of our personal motives. If you are one such, do, for heaven's sake, open your eyes to your gross ignorance and low propensities or be not surprised if one day you find yourself face to face with some powerful scoundrel who would not scruple to crush you in all possible ways. "Harm watch, harm catch." I am going to give you in practical form what constitute the real cause at the back of a "Magnetic" personality—that which when developed makes a god-like man of any human weakling.

This power is by no means the especial and peculiar possession of some divinely gifted individuals. *Everyone can cultivate it.* It is in you and needs vigorous stirring up as a condition of its awakening. There are some men who are born great; others are made so by certain unforeseen circumstances; a third class becomes great through conscious and intelligent effort.

Now, what are the causes behind Personal Influence?

(1) Some say that the right control of the Sex-Force or Celibacy is the cause.

(2) Others say that vegetarianism leads to it.

(3) Still others assert that it is physical energy and nerve force.

(4) A fourth class has it that there emanates a current of magnetism from the human body and influences everyone coming within its "Magnetic field".

Taking the last view point first, I should say, with certain other leading mental Scientists, that the human dynamic force is different from "magnetism" as the latter bears direct reference to the loadstone.

Again, my own personal observations as well as those of others prove conclusively that although "magnetic" personalities have remarkably well-disciplined and highly trained physical energies, it is rarely or never a huge gigantic physique with large, unsightly muscles that exerts this force. No, it is decidedly something other than mere physical energy and brute strength. A light, active, vigorous physique is desirable and any one can have it. Again, the principle value of a non-flesh diet lies in the fact that fruits, nuts, corn and vegetables are possessed of rhythmic qualities and go to build up a fine, sensitive physique capable of greater powers of endurance and sustained mental effort than the 'carcass' of any animal ever can. Matter does affect mind in the lower stages of organic evolution but the process is largely reversed as soon as CONSCIOUS evolution commences. Therefore vegetarianism, although highly commendable, from a strictly scientific point of view for the development of an active and energetic, refined organism, is by no means a rigid and indispensable necessity in this respect. In fact, some most "magnetic" individuate make 'graveyards of their stomachs' as a Mental Scientist puts it.

Lastly, Bramhacharya or Celibacy, as practised by Sannyasis in India, has a strictly spiritual significance although it certainly has much as everything to do with Personal Magnetism. To the average man I would say: "Strive for CONTINENCE, chastity and control in this direction." Do not emasculate, as that would be a waste of force. The stronger this force, the better. All Sannyasis learn consciously or unconsciously to transmute this energy into mental and spiritual force and generally their minds dwell on a plane of mental and spiritual effort where there cannot be even a breath of sensuality or grossness. They have gone beyond such things utterly; the same statement applies to all advanced thinkers, philosophers and workers, whether married or unmarried. To me the very name of philosophy carries with it an atmosphere of Chastity, Solemnity, and Divinity.

But although there is some measure of truth in all the above four statements, they all miss the real thing. The question resolves itself into this: "*What makes one man superior to another*?" The study of nature shows us that the higher form of intelligence controls the lower. All leaders of mankind, such as Napoleon, Alexander, etc., were clearly ahead of the times. But they strove for low things and their SUCCESS from our point of view is doubtful. Let us take higher ground. Buddha, Christ, Zoroaster, etc., etc., of ancient times and Vivekananda and a few others in modern times exhibited tremendous powers of influencing men. You study their lives and writings and try to find out just those things that constituted the basic cause of their heroic fibre.

If I were asked to sum up the secrets of their Power I would say:

1. "*Their Intelligence* and *Thought-Power*.

2. Awakened *Will-Power* and *Self-Control*."

1. It was by their intelligence that they could take fearless possession of the world, handle men and women easily, read human nature at a glance and "be all things to all men," *i.e..*, put their fingers direct on the spiritual, mental, and physical *necessities* of   widely   varying temperaments and help each right where he stood in the ladder of evolution.

2. It was by their developed thought-force that they drew the whole world to themselves. The positive thinker generates a force that draws all such as are *negative* to him. Nearly the whole world was negative to these Masters and hence felt attracted to them. *These were the human touchstones.*

3. It was by their strong, manly, marvelous Will-Power that they drove their suggestions into other minds and gained an immediate ascendency over whatever environments they were placed in. The whole man is summed up in his Will. Every other power in man is subservient to the Will. And say what you will, it is this power more than any other that we respect in others. It is the central staff in our character. Intelligence is the directive energy. Will-Power is the propulsive energy. And the latter when

wielded under the guidance of the former makes of man a veritable God.

4. It was by their unusual power of *Self-control* that they could stand square upon their feet and could remain unshaken by the waves of conflicting opinions and the hostile attacks that continually dashed up against them. *Master yourself*, i.e., your personal, relative and lower self, and beyond the shadow of a doubt, *the mastery of others is already yours.* But the world will teach you bitter lessons and rend you to pieces if you try consciously to control it while you are still a slave to your lower self. Be great. Strive for Perfection. So will you be recognized by others. And according to the transcendent energy of the highest law of our Being it is the consciousness of heights scaled, accomplishments achieved and consequent dawning of a Loftier Ideal upon our intellectual horizon that fills us with Strength and Peace rather than the recognition of our worth by others. It is a serious mistake to care for fame, praise and admiration. You get them only when you do not care for them in the least, when your soul has outgrown all such clinging to the relative in the light of *eternal thought*, when you have risen to the Absolute and learnt to read the meaning of the "LARGER WORLD" of life. Do not pass by this lightly. In it is the key to Peace, Power and Poise. All that is Real and Permanent, is on the plane of the Absolute.

Now we are drawing to the practical side of our Lesson. The four principal points, you will please remember, are: (1) Intelligence. (2) Thought-Force. (3) Will-Power. (4) Self-Control. You might feel surprised at my retailing this "ancient history" instead of teaching you how to approach a man, make him your slave and command him to fall down at your feet and do your bidding. Perhaps you expected me to tell you how to sail through the air, pass through solid walls, materialize and dematerialize at will and like Appolonius of Tyana vanish in the flash of an eye from the court of Ionysius and appear elsewhere at a distance of 19,000 miles at the same moment. No, no. I will take it for granted that you are made of different stuff and *an earnest seeker after the truth.* If you strive to build yourself on the basis of the simple principles as laid down in this series of lessons you will in time grow into the Higher Self and at last become one with it. Moreover, your daily life will be the Occasion for the practical application of these principles, thus enabling you to pursue your way through life calmly, earnestly, independently and with the quiet dignity of a man "who knows what he is about". I cannot and would not speak of "get-rich-quick" methods of self-development because they are the veriest rot imaginable.

Now then: (1) Intelligence and (2) Thought-Force are the natural results of an organized brain.

Concentration is the key to such development. Concentration has been fully explained in Lesson No. 1. By the constant exercise of concentration, objectively and subjectively, in your daily life you will in a short time become conscious of growing Strength. The exercises I give you in this lesson on Self-Control, Will-Culture and Memory-Culture if gone through with perseverance will further develop Concentrative ability. In fact, this entire series of lessons will call for Effort and Concentration. "Rome was not built in a day"— nor can you achieve real greatness in a few months. No. All I can do is to indicate the line and the nature of the effort required of you and if clearly followed, Progress and Growth will commence from the first day. In connection with this, a little digression would be necessary. The Occultist says: Nature, unaided, fails. The purposiveness of Deity, manifesting in nature an evolution, is present in all individual centers but it has the way to full expression opened out to itself only when the more evolved centers of life consciously cooperate with it. Evolution is started and carried only by the creation of centers within the GREAT CONSCIOUSNESS and by preserving and enlarging or expanding these centers. So long as the race had not reached "SELF-CONSCIOUSNESS" (see Yoga Lessons) the sub-conscious forces of nature had entire control over evolutionary processes, but this stage was reached by the race according to the LAW OF AVERAGES in the seventeenth century and you are now expected to take your progress in your hands and consciously direct your inner forces along such lines as best correspond to the stage of your growth. So independent study and steady thinking form the secrets of a keen and broad intelligence. You will always find that the man who is more powerful than yourself and moves you at his will has an intelligence and understanding far superior to yours and he can read your whole nature as he would an open book, although you find him quite beyond your depth. Learn to regard earnestly the workings of different mentalities around you. Become a student of human nature. To you, each man ought to be only a partial expression of his mind. Examine closely into the motives acting behind each personality. Learn to respond more quickly to the *Thoughts* and *Feelings* of a man than to his outer speech and action. The latter are objective expressions of the subjective self. The study of Phrenology and Physiognomy are good things to start with in your efforts to acquire knowledge of human nature. *Mind is One* and at the same time, *Many*. Subjectively, it is ONE. Objectively; many. So by looking *impartially* into "yourself" in the calm light of the intellect and through silent introspection, you will always find a clue to the working bases of other minds. Each man is a puzzle and most of all are *YOU* a puzzle unto yourself. Solve either and you have solved both. "MAN, KNOW THYSELF."

THE MYSTERY OF THE WILL-FORCE.

Will-Force is the power of Re-action. It can render all the other mental functions *active* or *passive*. It is the DETERMINATIVE faculty and is affected most of all by the JUDGMENT. On the lower plane of mind, Will-Power manifests as Desire and is reciprocally influenced by outside attractions as well as repulsions. On this plane the Will is not free. But when it draws the volition for externalizing itself from *Within* in the light of the Higher Reason, then indeed is it *Will-Power. On the material the human will is a slave; on the spiritual plane it is the sovereign. It may then be called the "awakened" will*. It is my conviction that the eternal crossing of swords between the Determinists and the Libertarians can be set at rest only by a right understanding of the *spiritual* makeup of man, otherwise the arguments of both sets of thinkers are equally strong. Each side has got hold of half the truth, but requires the reconciling light of transcendental Psychology in order to enable us to see the *whole* truth as it is. However, the point I am driving at is that your will is free only when it is *self-determined* i.e., when it has risen above the impulses of the Lower Personal Self and acts under the direction of the Higher Impersonal Self_. In order to fix this most important truth in your mind, let us give you a brief idea of the "I AM" consciousness. Do not pass this by as so much dry rot. No one will ever or can ever manifest genuine Will-Force of a distinctly spiritual type who does not understand the "I AM" consciousness. So please listen attentively and think over the following.

THE "I AM" CONSCIOUSNESS.

If you just turn in and examine the report of your consciousness regarding the *self*-dwelling within, you will become conscious of the "I". But if you press your examination a little closer you will find that this "I" may be split up into two distinct aspects which, while working in unison and conjunction, may nevertheless be set apart in thought. There is an "I" function and there is a "me" function and these mental twins develop distinct phenomena. The first is the "MASCULINE" principle; the second is the "FEMININE" principle. Other terms used in current writings on New Psychology are Conscious Mind, Active Mind, Voluntary Mind, Objective Mind and so forth. These all refer to the "I" principle. And the "me" form of mind corresponds to the Sub-Conscious Mind, Passive Mind, Involuntary Mind, Subjective Mind and so on. Ninety-nine p. c. of humanity mean this "me" when they say "I". Now let us examine what this "me" implies. It consists largely of our consciousness, of our body and physical sensations as associated with touch, taste, smell, sight and hearing. The consciousness of some of us is largely bound up in the physical and carnal side of life. We "live there." There are some men who consider their "clothes" too as being a part of themselves. But as consciousness rises in the scale of evolution, man begins to "dissociate" his idea of "me" from the body and he begins to regard his body as a beloved companion and as "belonging to" him. He then identifies himself with his mental states, emotions, feelings, likes and dislikes, habits, qualities and characteristics. But, by and by, he begins to realize how even these moods also are subject to change, born and die and are subject to the Principles of Rhythm and Polarity. He realizes faintly that he can change them by an effort of will and "transmute" them into mental states of an exactly opposite nature. Then he again begins to "dissociate" himself from his emotions and feelings and at last through mental analysis, introspection and concentration, he sets them apart into the "not I" collection. He begins *then* to realize that he is something *above* his body and emotions. So also with the intellectual functions. The intellectual man is very apt to think that although his *physical* and *emotional* selves are something different from him and under his control, *still his intellect is himself.* This is the stage of "Self-Consciousness". "I control my body and emotions." But as consciousness unfolds intellectual man finds that he can practically stand aside and see (mentally, of course) his mind going through various processes of intellection. Study of Psychology and Logic will enable you to see how all your intellectual processes may be held at arm's length, examined, analysed, labelled and discussed quite with the same ease as the professor talks of a solid, liquid and aciform substances in his laboratory. So at last he finds that even the wonderful powers of the Intellect must go into the "not I" collection. This is almost as far as the average man can realize. You can realize and say "I am not the body, not the emotions, not the intellect." Therefore you see, that side of consciousness which is the sum-total of your physical, emotional and intellectual functions comprises the "me" or Feminine or Passive mental principle. That which can separate itself in thought from all the above is the "I" or the Masculine Function. But another step must be taken. That which you have been taught to regard as the Spiritual Consciousness (see "Spiritual Consciousness") will also eventually go into the "Not-I" or "me" collection. In brief, the spiritual mind may be said to comprise all that is GOOD, NOBLE and GREAT in the field of consciousness. It is the "Super-Conscious" mind, just now. But, mark this, when through further evolution, the "I" has mastered this field of consciousness also and is able to regard it as being the last of the "me" collections, then it will lose its sense of *relativity* and *separation* and the real individuality, the "I AM" consciousness, will have been realized. What do I mean? This "I AM" is not the petulant self-assertion of the relative ego. "I" but really means GOD CONSCIOUSNESS as perfect Existence, perfect Knowledge or perfect Bliss. It means the realization of an Infinite and Eternal Self or

Individuality. "He that has lost the self has gained the SELF". Here is the explanation: this little self or "I" so long as it is attached to the PERSONALITY which is the product of the "me" consciousness is bound down to the relative plane. It can think only through only one brain, enjoy through one body and such happiness as it gets is transitory, short-lived and impermanent because this world of relative existence is itself essentially changeable. It is permanent only in its impermanence. So long as the "I" thinks and while only for the benefits of its personal self, both thinking and willing are limited and not free. But when it has succeeded in joining itself to the Spiritual mind and works for, aspires after the Larger Self—the "I AM"—it has to renounce or "disattach" itself from the personal self and work under the guidance of the impersonal Higher Self. "I refuse to be contained within my hat and boots," said Walt Whitman. When the Vedantist says "Aham Brahmasmi"—"I am the absolute"—he does not mean this lower "I". No, no. He is not built that way. For him the moorings of self-consciousness are out. He has lost all sense of his particular relative "I" and has *one-d* himself with the absolute "I AM"—the impersonal, intangible, immortal, omnipotent Self of and over all. This "I am" is Spirit or Atman. There can be but one Individuality—that of the Absolute. It becomes objectively expressed in man as Cosmic Consciousness. Subjectively it is God. Now then you have an idea of the "I am" Consciousness. Hold fast to it. It is your real,

Larger Self. In the understanding and the exercise of the Will-Power the "I" or the Positive Mental Principle is the chief factor. To use the one you must understand the other. Will is a Soul-Power. This "I"—as I have explained it above—is negative to the "I AM" or God—both meaning the same thing. It is positive in relation to the Higher Self. This "I" is the future promise of the "I AM". It is true it shall lose itself in finding its Self, but so does the child when it grows into full manhood. Christ was one with his Father-in-Heaven (i.e., on the spiritual plane) and therefore he could still the waves and raise the dead. Yet just you examine the nature of Lord Christ's Will-Force. Think of his constant retirement into the Silence in order to obtain inspiration for his work in the objective universe. Again, note his utter indifference to and absolute control over his personal self. Did he care whether his body would live or die? Did he live for the enjoyments of the flesh? Did he "play to the gallery" and act and speak for any worldly gain or low considerations? No! He had forgotten the interests of the flesh in his earnest enthusiasm in the cause of the Eternal Spirit. He was not moved by any dammed sense of prudence and caution. He drew the "Motives" that energized his Will-Power in the life of Action from *Within*. Nothing from outside, nothing from the world of lower attractions could in the least swerve his inner determination or unbalance his brain. Do you or can you prepare yourself to follow in his steps? Then my first point and the most infallible method of awakening your Will-Power is this:

(a) Teach Thy Will to "Resist and Renounce." Strengthen your Will-Power by Renunciation. By Resistance is not meant outer resistance or aggressiveness. I find that all the modern teachers of Hypnotism advise their students to develop Will-Power by exercising it upon others. This is placing the cart before the horse. We Hindus know better. No; by Resistance to and Repression of your lower Desire-Nature is meant letting the more difficult choice exercise its compelling and restraining power over the easier one. Says Sister Nivedita: "The Indian ideal is that man whose lower mind is so perfectly under control that he can at any moment plunge into the thought-ocean and remain there at will without the least possibility of a sudden break and unexpected return to the life of the senses." Yes, your interests should be within and not without. *You must rise above all personal impulse.* Even in this world you find that men of distinction, fame and honor have achieved recognition by practicing a little *self-denial*, which is a "milder" form of absolute Renunciation as practiced by true Sanyasis. The man who can work at his aim with perseverance and denies himself the mess of pottage of present indulgence in view of some future gain develops Will-Power. So in training your Will to 'resist', you must, as a first step, sternly refuse to indulge impulses, desires and tendencies not in consonance with the dictates of your Higher Self.

You must actually go out of your way and "deny" yourself the little or great "comforts" to which you are or have been accustomed. The strongest-willed man is he who has the greatest control over his inclinations, and who can 'force' himself to do such things as he is naturally most inclined to do. This is a characteristic which cannot be developed in a day. There are some children and even grown-up men and women who mistake their 'obstinacy' for Will-Power. They want a thing and when they do not get it they tear their hair, gnash their teeth, stamp their feet and fly into a terrible passion. Since people think that these uncontrolled creatures are strong-willed while all that you could say about them is that *they are utter slaves to their desires.* You must practice self-denial in fifty different ways and force yourself to do certain things, 'little and big,' every day purely for developing this power of Resistance. No short-cut to this. Some children develop it unconsciously by 'forcing' themselves to study when they might play, and by applying themselves to such studies as are dry and uninteresting to them they thus practice voluntary Concentration. Practice self-denial in every possible way. Cut off such luxuries as you think "you must have." "Take a cold bath when you would prefer a warm one. Arise promptly in the morning. Make yourself call upon people you have avoided. Stand up in a street car when you would prefer sitting; walk when it is convenient to ride. Make engagements with yourself and keep them. Promise yourself that when you see something to be done you will spring at once to it however strong may be the inclination to put it off awhile" and back of it all let there be the auto-suggestion: "*I am doing all these hard things in order to build up my Will-Power and each time 'I' succeed in forcing 'my mind' to do a thing or not to do it I make the next victory easier and my Will-Power stronger.*" Of course the above is only a hint as to your line of practice.

(*b*) You must not give yourself such hard tasks of Self-Development as might be too heavy and beyond the present strength of your Will. In denying yourself you develop self-control. In forcing yourself to do certain things you develop powers of Self-Expression. In one the Will moves along negative lines. In the other along positive lines. Both are necessary. The man who cannot control and command himself can never develop and express Himself. But be sure to begin with easy things and then as you gain in confidence you may attempt more difficult feats.

(*c*) The faculties of Courage and Confidence are essentially important. Nothing weakens the will so much as Fear and lack of Self-Confidence. Self-Confidence is not blustering self-conceit. That within you which says "I CAN" when calmly and doggedly backed by your "I Will" when deliberately translated into action develops Will-Force and commands startling results.

(*d*) Always hold these words before your passive Mind:

1. Earnestness. 2. Determination. 3. Courage. 4. Confidence. 5. Stick-to-it-ive-ness. 6. Patience. 7. I can and I will.

(*e*) The tendency of the Masculine function of your mind to "I" is towards giving, expressing or projecting energy; that of the Feminine is towards generating and creating mental progeny such as thoughts, mental energy, new habits, etc. It is why the Feminine Principle has been called the "mental womb" by ancient philosophers. It comprises also the faculty of Imagination. The Masculine function does the work of the 'Will' in its varied phases. The Feminine function receives impressions and generates mental offspring in the form of new thoughts, ideas, concepts, thought-habits and so forth. Its powers of creative energy are strikingly marvelous and have been proved and attested to in Psychological experiments conducted by the best known mental scientists of the day. *But "positive" mental energy must be projected by the 'I' into the Passive Mind through concentration, suggestion and willing before the latter can be started to work along any line of creative effort.* This suggestion may be given by you to your sub-conscious mind or it may come as an outer impression. Unless you control your Passive Mind, it is sure to be controlled by others. Then you are a slave. Now in cultivating the above seven qualities, you should take up *one* word at a time and let the outer form sink into your mind. Place yourself in a relaxed and passive condition. Close your eyes and picture the *form* of the word to yourself, for instance, D-E-T-E-R-M-I-N-A-T-I-O-N. Employ the Imagination and visualize mentally. This done, *i.e.*, when the word-picture is well photographed upon your mind and fastened in place, your next step will be to picture yourself the Ideas, qualities, physical and mental characteristics, etc., associated with the word. Your third step is to calmly, concentrated and confidently command your Passive Mind to generate that quality. Remember, your mind will at first rebel, but a very little persistence will lead to complete success. Repeat the auto-suggestions daily at the same time. See that it manifests in Action. Act it out as often as possible. Of course your efforts will be imperfect to begin with, but, never mind, go ahead, keeping firm hold on your "I can and I will" in spite of all things and success is quite certain. Once you have developed these seven qualities, you can do anything.

(*f*) Do not let your friends or anyone—no matter who!—deflect you from your resolutions. "Let not thy right hand knows what thy left hand does." Talk never. Let results show. The Lord has hidden himself best and His work is wonderful beyond compare! Your very friends and relatives will spit upon you for lacking any of these qualities. Do not ever impose your will upon others, but never let others to impose upon you against the sanction of your own judgment. In fact, none can unless you are a weakling and fickle-minded.

(*g*) Frequent the company of chaste, strong-willed men and you cannot but grow strong.

(*h*) Read Literature on this subject and obtain all possible aid through Knowledge.

(*i*) If your faculty of imagination and idealism are undeveloped, cultivate them, because it is these two that make a god of a man. Philosophers, scholars, poets and musicians have them well-developed. But where imagination is uncontrolled by higher reason and where idealism is not backed by a strong will, there you have the idle 'dreamer of dreams' and such a state of mind is reprehensible and pitiable indeed!

(*j*) Will-Power grows by faith in one's ability by exercise; by devotion to the UNCONDITIONED SPIRIT.

(*k*) In your efforts to develop Will-Power, be not afraid that your health will break down. In fact, Perfect Health is the result of a perfect Will. Deny the power of disease and weakness over yourself. "*I can never be ill. My body is my slave. It shall always manifest perfect health.*" Convince your passive mind—which has charge of your body—of this by repeated commands, demands and assertions. Always think of your body as being as strong as adamant. Never talk of either health or disease or weakness. You must be above caring for these. They are your Natural rights. Only when you lower yourself they have power to trouble you. Go beyond the lower self.

Your business is to care for the Higher-Self—that in which "You" live, move, and have your being. Also teach and train your Will to move along negative lines of self-repression as well as along positive lines of Self-Expression. Balance both. The former precedes the latter. Now I will pass on to the subject of SELF-CONTROL, with the distinct understanding that Self-Control and Will-Power are inextricably bound up in each other. You Get the real "practical work" in the endeavor for Self-Control.

SELF-CONTROL.

Rightly has it been remarked that is easy to talk of and write upon this subject but most difficult to possess it. Perfect Self-Control means infinite power. Only the Buddas and the Christs of this World manifested Perfect Self-Control. "Anything short of the absolute control of thought, word and deed is only sowing wild oats," said Vivekananda. It is with no little diffidence that I approach this subject as whoever handles this subject is rightly culpable as being a "Do-as-I-say-and-not-as-I-do" class of writers. Still you can make appreciable progress in this direction by mastering these instructions, going through the exercises and last but most important by "carrying the principles in your mind" and applying them as far as you can in your daily life. Nothing is more conducive to rapid growth and development as the making of the "little and big" affairs in your work-a-day life, the occasion for the practical expression and conscious translation of your ideals. We all are guilty of a serious mistake in setting apart our higher ideals for regular 'practice' hours and leading a life of low and quite different ideals in our ordinary life. The natural process, as you can see, is to LIVE OUT your highest ideals every minute of your life. Nothing is more important than the daily occupation of a man and if he fails to bring his ideals right into these little things, then Success will ever elude him. A mental scientist has summed up the entire secret of Character-Building in this valuable advice on Objective Concentration: the simple task of mental concentration on whatever task, business or profession a man is engaged in is the beginning of the mastery which is the perfection of Objective Concentration. Whatever you are doing be master of your work. If you are a cobbler mend shoes in a perfect manner; if a barber keep your razors and scissors in a state that will excite the admiration of your customers; if a tailor make the coat fit like a glove; if a clerk keep your accounts in apple-pie order; if a builder scorn your jerry-brother; if a singer enchant the listener with a concord of sweet sounds; if an actor enter into the spirit of the character and make the play-goer feel that

"All the world's a stage And all the men and women merely players, They have their exits and their entrance. And one man in his time plays many parts."

If a leader in any department of thought or action, remember that if to you much is given, from you also much is required, for the responsibility of the lives and happiness of your fellows rests heavy on your shoulders, whether you know it or not and thousands may secretly curse your incapacity and bungling. It is infinitely better to be a good cobbler than a bad ruler.

I believe the above advice if followed conscientiously by you would go to make you really fit for initiation into the more advanced stages of mastery. Take it to heart by all means. Be convinced, the man who looks for quick results and a royal road to the mastery of Mental Science breaks down in frequent despair at apparent failures and neglects his daily work will never go far. In fact, his very impatience will lead to failure. No individual life is fully rounded out unless some useful work forms part of it. The Yogi who has renounced the world has already done his work and is ahead of the times. The real hermit and the saint are the Pillars of Strength on which this world stands. I cannot repeat this too often. The mere fact of their breathing the same atmosphere as you is a benediction and an inestimable boon unto the race.

PRELIMINARY STEPS.

"The first requisite," says Mr. Atkinson, "of concentering is the ability to shut out outside thoughts, sights and sounds; to conquer inattention; to obtain perfect control over the body and mind. The body must be brought under the control of the mind; the mind under the direct control of the Will. The Will is strong enough, but the mind needs strengthening by being brought under the direct influence of the will. The mind, strengthened by the impulse of the will, becomes a much more powerful projector of thought vibrations than otherwise and the vibrations have much greater force and effect."

The first four exercises are meant to train the mind to readily obey the commands of the mind. Take them in the privacy of your own room and never talk of them to others. Also do not let their apparent simplicity lead you to neglect them. If you are one of those empty-brained men who go about talking of their exercises hoping in this way to win praise, you will never succeed. Be serious, earnest and sincere in your work. Give up, once forever, all fickle-mindedness and learn to accumulate Power in silence and through work. Prayer gives you strength to "work"—the answer comes from your Larger Self—which is the Spirit of God "brooding" over all and pouring strength into all. But do not fly in the face of DEITY by expecting it to "do the work" for you while you go about loafing after offering your prayer. Nonsense. That man prays who works constantly, silently, patiently, unceasingly and intelligently.

Exercise 1.

Sit still; relax your body all over and then neck, chest, and head held in a straight line; legs crossed one under the other and weight of the body resting easily upon the ribs; right hand on right leg, left hand on left leg. There should not be a single movement of the muscles in any part of the body. Mind, you must avoid all rigidness and tension of the body. There should not be the least strain on muscles. You should be able to "relax" completely. Start with 5 minutes. Continue till you can accomplish the 5 minutes sitting without any conscious effort, increase to 15 minutes which is about all you need. The aim is to give you absolute dominion over all involuntary muscular movements. It is also an ideal "rest-cure" after fatiguing physical and mental exercise or exertion. The principal thing is "STILLNESS" and you can, if you like, practice it even sitting on a chair or anywhere else; the idea is one of "relaxation" and physical and mental quietude. Let not the apparent simplicity of this exercise deceive you. It is not so very easy after all. You will find that by concentrating the mind upon a particular train of thoughts or ideas or by joining the mind to the Larger Self, you can easily lose all idea of the body and thus maintain this stillness for a considerable length of time. Genius, inspiration and intuition are more or less the scientific and psychological results of self-forgetfulness. "When he sits down to meditate," it was said of Vivekananda, "in 10 minutes he becomes quite unconscious of the body although it may be black with mosquitoes." Do you understand now? Absolute physical self-forgetfulness is essential to deep concentration. Dr. Fahnestock called it the "STATUVOLIC" condition or that state in which the Will-Power is really active and the 'outer-self' is totally in abeyance and forgotten.

Exercise 2.

Cultivate a self-poised attitude and demeanor in your everyday life. Avoid a tense, strained, nervous, fidgety manner and an over-anxious appearance. Be easy, self-possessed and dignified in your bearing. Be courteous, thoughtful and quiet. Mental exercise and Will-Culture will enable you to acquire the proper carriage and demeanor. Stop swinging your feet and moving your hands or rocking yourself backwards in your chair while talking or sitting. Stop biting your nails, chewing your moustaches, rolling your tongue in your mouth or any other unnecessary movement such as may have become "second nature" with you while studying, reading or writing. Never twitch or jerk your body. Never wink your eyes or look blank. Train yourself to stand sudden and loud noises with equanimity and composure. Such things betray lack of control. Do not let anything outside (or even within you) disturb your composure. When engaged in conversation let your speech be calm and measured and your voice well-controlled and even. A certain degree of reserve should always be observed. In short, keep yourself well under control on all occasions. You can acquire this poise by always carrying the thoughts of "Firmness," "Self-Control", and "Self-Respect" in your mind and letting these express themselves in your outward bearing. Avoid bluster, self-assertion, gossip, levity or light talk, too much laughter, excitement and so forth. Too much laughter weakens the will. Be a quiet, earnest-thinking being. Be serious. Regard "solitude" as the greatest medium of self-development.

Exercise 3.

Fill a wine glass full of water and taking the glass between the fingers, extend arm directly in front of you. Fix your eyes upon the glass and endeavor to hold your arm so steady that no quiver will be noticeable. Commence with one minute exercise and increase until the 5 minutes limit is reached. Alternate right and left arms. Increase to 15 minutes.

Exercise 4.

Sit erect in your chair, with your head up, chin out and shoulders back. Raise your right arm until it is level with your shoulders, pointing to the right. Turn your head and fix your gaze on your hand and hold the arm perfectly steady for one minute. Repeat with left arm. Increase the time gradually to 5 minutes. The palms of the hands should be turned downwards.

The following exercises are meant to aid you in getting under control, such mental faculties will produce voluntary movements.

Exercise 5.

Sit in front of a table, placing your hands upon the table, the fists clinched and lying with the back of the hand upon the table, the thumb being doubled over the fingers. Fix your gaze upon the fist for a while and then slowly extend the thumb, keeping your whole attention fixed upon the act, just as if it was of the greatest importance. Then slowly extend your first finger, then your second and so on, until they are all open and extended. Then reverse the process, closing first the little finger and continuing the closing until the fist is again in its original position, with the thumb closed over the fingers. Repeat with left hand. Continue this exercise 5 times at a sitting, then increase to 10 times. Don't forget to keep your attention closely fixed upon the finger movements. That is the main point.

Exercise 6.

Place the fingers of one hand between the fingers of the other, leaving the thumbs free. Then slowly twirl the thumbs one over the other, with a circular motion. Be sure to keep the attention firmly fixed upon the end of the thumbs.

N.B. Exercises Nos. 3, 4, 5 and 6 have been culled (with slight modifications by me) from the works of Yogi Ramacharaka.

Exercise 7.

Forty-eight hours after the full moon in each month, go by yourself into a darkened chamber and quietly concentrate your mind upon one thing. Do this as long as possible without allowing other thoughts to enter your mind. At first you will find that your thoughts will fly from one thing to another and it will be hard for you to accomplish this, but by continued practice you will be able to think of one thing for a long time. This should be continued for 5 nights in succession and one hour each night.

Exercise 8.

Go out into the open air each evening when the sky is clear and see how many stars you can count without allowing any other thoughts to enter your mind. The more stars you can count without thinking of anything the greater the degree of development produced. Quite an interesting exercise.

Exercise 9.

Take 12 ordinary pebbles. Place them in your left hand. Then with your right hand pick up one pebble, hold it at arm's length and concentrate your mind thereupon without allowing other thoughts for full 60 seconds. So with all the pebbles. Then start picking up with left hand. Do this for one hour daily.

Exercise 10.

Concentrate your mind determinedly upon someone at a distance without allowing other thoughts. Will that he do get strong, healthy and spiritual. Get up a mental picture of your subject as if sitting before you. Then give earnest, positive, forceful suggestions to his sub-conscious mind. Will that he get into sympathy with you, write you on the subject and earnestly co-operate with you in his spiritual regeneration. Do it calmly and earnestly.

Exercise 11.

Get some moistened sand spread over the surface about a yard square. Make it perfectly smooth. Then with your index finger draw any characters or pictures in the sand. For instance, a square, a triangle or any other figure. Fasten your gaze upon this figure. Concentrate your mind calmly thereupon and will that the thought-form so created by your concentration be transmitted to someone (whom you know to be sensitive to your will). Do this for 15 minutes daily at the same time till your subject gets the impression. Ask him to sit relaxed at the same time in the *silence* in a receptive mental attitude. Face the direction, North, South, East or West in which you send your thought. Imagine a psychic wire connecting you with your subject and aim straight. Remember, the Will-Power is represented in symbology by a straight line because it goes straight to its mark.

Exercise 12.

Every night before retiring, concentrate upon your passive mind: "*When I get up in morning, my Will-power and Thought-Force will have increased. I expect you to bring about a thorough change in my Will-Force. It will gain in vigour, resolution, firmness and confidence. It must grow strong, strong, strong.*" Project these positive suggestions into your subjective self earnestly, confidently and concentrated. You will progress quickly by leaps and bounds. Every morning shall find you stronger and full of vim, sap and energy. Persevere, persevere. In following up such ideals to a successful conclusion you must have an (i) overpowering desire; (ii) a strong belief in your ability to accomplish anything; (iii) an invincible determination not a backboneless 'I will try to'; (iv) earnest expectation. This is an important and an infallible method in Will-development.

Exercise 13.

Go by yourself into a room where you will not be disturbed. At the beginning 'relax' all over. Then count from one to ten without allowing any other thoughts. As soon as you accomplish this, your mind is in a receptive state. Concentrate as before and order your sub-conscious self to evolve a strong, infallible memory. Form your own auto-suggestions.

Exercise 14.

Pick out half a dozen unfamiliar faces. Vividly impress them upon your subjective mind. Then recall them at least once each day for full one year, each day impressing at least one more new face. Should you find you are forgetting any of your older faces, do not add new ones but firmly fix the other old faces in your mind through concentration. This is a very interesting exercise. Memory belongs to the sub-conscious mind, remember.

Exercise 15.

Concentrate the mind on a paragraph in some holy book and commit to memory. Learn by heart one paragraph daily taking care not to forget the old ones. In time, you will improve wonderfully.

Exercise 16.

People with weak memories always lack concentrative ability. Concentration is the key to all mind-power. You will find the above exercises quite 'tedious' and monotonous. But you can train your 'attention' only by giving it trivial and 'dry' exercises. The strong will can cope with the most 'monotonous' and uninteresting tasks without experiencing fatigue. You must set yourself such tasks as might seem like 'work' to your attention. Remember, the effort required to concentrate attention voluntarily on uninteresting, dry and monotonous works strengthens and develops Will-Power and gives you 'mental muscle.' You will thereby acquire firm control over mind and body and be 'Master' over your lower impulses. Power over self will express outwardly as power over others. If you can control yourself, you will find no difficulty in impressing your will on others. But, mark you, this sacred power should be used only to elevate, stimulate and strengthen others. Try your Will upon your personality in all possible ways and be satisfied with nothing short of perfect control. The absolute mastery of 'self' ought to be your aim. I have given you the real secrets. You must exercise your own ingenuity and intelligence in utilising them towards your Self-development. I leave you to finish the fight for yourself. Get up and start in to work at your task from to-day and not to-morrow. Back of all efforts, always have this positive incentive and auto-suggestion:

"THIS IS TO DEVELOP MY WILL-POWER AND NO TEMPORARY PAIN CAN EQUAL THE POWER AND HAPPINESS ARISING OUT OF SELF-CONTROL."

Get firm control over your emotions. Use this natural force but be not used by it. Control over speech will lead to Emotion-control. Always talk to the point. Cultivate silence. Repress volubility. Be brief in speech and writing. Keep a cool head. Be level-headed and concentrative.

GLEANINGS FROM PROFESSOR JAMES ON THE LAW OF HABIT.

An acquired habit, from the physiological point of view, is nothing but a new pathway of discharge formed in the brain, by which certain incoming currents ever often tend to escape.

The great thing is to make our nervous system our ally instead of our enemy.—Guard against ways that are likely to be disadvantageous to us, as we should guard against the plague.

The more of the details of our daily life we can hand over to the effortless custody of automatism, the more our higher powers of mind will be set free for their own proper work. There is no more miserable human being than one in whom nothing is habitual but indecision and for whom (every act) the time of rising and going to bed, the beginning of every bit of work, are subjects for express volitional deliberation.

Maxim I. In the acquisition of a new thought or the leaving off of an old one we must take care to launch ourselves with as strong and decided initiative as possible.

Maxim II. Never suffer an exception to occur until the new habit is securely rooted in your life.

Each lapse is like letting fall a ball of string which one is carefully winding up; a single slip means more than a great many turns will wind again.

Continuity of training is the great means of making the nervous system act infallibly right. It is necessary above all things never to lose a battle. Every gain on the wrong side undoes the effect of many conquests on the right.

The essential precaution is to so regulate the opposing powers that the one may have a series of uninterrupted success, until repetition has fortified it to such a degree as to enable it to cope with the opposition under any circumstances.

The need of securing success at the outset is imperative. To be habitually successful is the thing.

Be careful not to give the will such a task as to insure its defeat at the outset, but provided one can stand it, a sharp period of suffering, and then a free time is the best to aim at, whether in giving up the opium habit or in simply changing one's hours of rising or of work.

It is surprising how soon a desire will die of inanition if it be never fed.

Without unbroken advance there is no such thing as accumulation of the ethical forces possible, and to make this possible and to exercise and habituate us in it is the sovereign blessing of regular work. Maxim III. Seize the very first possible opportunity to act on every resolution you make and on every emotional prompting you may experience in the direction of habits you aspire to gain.

It is not the moment of their forming but in the moment of their producing motor effects, that resolves and aspirations communicate the new 'set' to the brain.

The actual presence of the practical opportunity alone furnishes the fulcrum upon which the lever can rest, by means of which the moral will may multiply its strength and raise itself aloft. He who had no solid ground to press against will never get beyond the stage of empty gesture making.

When a resolve or a fine glow of feeling is allowed to evaporate without bearing practical fruit, it is a waste and a chance lost; it works so as positively to hinder future resolutions and emotions from taking the normal path of discharge.

If we let our emotions evaporate, they get in a way of evaporating.

WORSHIP OF THE TERRIBLE.

The attitude of the soul which is not to be baffled by the lower nature or the "Personal Self" should be to seek Death and not life, to hurl oneself upon the sword's point and become one with the terrible. Those who are commissioned by the Lord to bear aloft the torch of spirit are fated to see every joy of the senses turn to ashes and crushing blows upon their eyes to the unsubstantially of the relative life of Maya.

The lion when stricken to the heart gives out his loudest roar,
When smitten on the head the cobra lifts its hood
And the majesty of the Soul comes out only when a man is wounded to his
depths.

The Western ideal is to be doing: the Eastern to be suffering. The perfect life would be a harmony between (selfless or non-attached) doing and suffering. Worship the terrible. Worship Death, for its own sake; despair for its own sake; pain for its own sake. Yet this is not the coward's or the suicide's or the weakling's morbid love of Death, but it is the cry of the philosopher who has sounded everything to its depths and knows intensely the vanity of the desire for happiness on the relative plane of limitations. Remember the triumphant cry of St. Francis of Assisi: "WELCOME, SISTER DEATH!" "Be witness"—of all that goes on but be not entangled. Reserve to yourself the power to remain unattached at all times. Accept nothing however pleasant, if it conceals a fetter into thy Soul. At a word stand ready to sever any connection that gives a hint of soul-bondage. Keep thy mind clear. Keep thy will pure. Attain the Impersonal Standpoint, O you man! there alone canst thou quench thy thirst for happiness never on the plane of personal. Who and what dies and is reborn?—Your lower self, your personality.

"Sometimes naked, sometimes mad,
Now as a scholar, again as a fool
Here a rebel, there a saint,
Thus they appear on the earth
—the Perfect Ones. Paramhamsas"—Viveka Chudamani.

If you accept the report of the senses as final, you will say "soul for nature"—but if you can gain the spiritual point of view, you will say "no-nature for soul." Evolution, devolution and involution are all in nature and will go on cyclically and eternally. All this is merely due to the wish of the soul to manifest itself. But such expression can come only when the soul lives on its plane. Say "Money is my slave, not I." Say "Nature is my slave, not I". Give up life, give up body, give up all desire for enjoyment on the relative plane. So shall you transcend all limitation. Your real nature is Infinite and Absolute. Only when you lower your nature by limiting it to the "particular self," do you become bound and unhappy. On the relative plane, you are a slave to the pair of opposites—life and death, pleasure and pain, and so on. Here is limitation. Here you are a slave to competition, and "Survival of the Fittest" is the law. Be not blinded by the flashing light of the glare of modern civilization. Every morsel you eat is ground out of your brother's blood. Slave to a breath of air, slave to food, slave to life, slave to Death, slave to a word of praise, slave to a word of blame—"Slave—Slave—Slave"—that is your condition. The Soul cannot stoop to any compromise. It refuses to conquer nature by obedience. It will conquer nature by renouncing the body and by knowing itself. Find thyself bodiless. Power felt within is soul; without, nature. "We must crush Law (nature) and become outlaws."

"Deliver thou thyself, by thyself
Ah, do not let thyself sink
For thou art thyself thy greatest friend
And thyself (the relative 'I') thy greatest enemy."

This, student, is not the ravings of a lunatic. It is the secret of SAT-CHIT-ANANDA—eternal existence, knowledge and bliss. Attainment of perfection means absolute Freedom. Do you or would you know the meaning of Life? It is the search after *Sat-chit-ananda*. But man is trying to realise this Perfect Existence in the transitory things of the earth-plane. Only when he knows that not attachment to the things of the "world, the flesh and the devil" but renunciation of same and the bringing of the Impersonal Ideal into his everyday life would lead him to it, then Maya will have fulfilled its purpose—which is to show man his divinity. "Kill out the desire for life. Kill out Ambition. Kill out desire for comfort; yet work as those who love life. Respect life as those who are ambitious. Be happy as those are who live for happiness."

So says Mabel Collins in the *Light on the Path*. Yes, you must work constantly, train your intellect, develop your personality but do not do all this for your own personal self but for the Higher Self, The BRAHMAN, Eternal—to manifest through. As soon as you lose this viewpoint your personal strivings end in Pain and Disappointment. Work as hard as the ambitious man and the lover of pleasures but remember your actions are inspired by different motives. Here Spirit is the director.

"To the work thou hast the right, O Partha, but not to the fruits thereof"—*Gita*. All clinging to results leads to degeneration. The soul should cling to nothing. All work and all effort must be dedicated unto the Higher Self. When you care for the results you are only worshipping the lower self. Hence the value of selfless labour, thus the maya-fascinated mind is purified and de-hypnotised and we attain to the emergence of the personal into the Impersonal. Either say "I am thou, O Lord!" and thus out at the root of the lower "I" and destroy it for ever or say "I am nothing, O Eternal One! thou art everything" and thereby lose the lower into the Higher. The first is for the Gnani—the second for the Bhakti Yogi. Both mean the same thing. Love everyone but do not depend upon the love of any one. Give everything. Take nothing. Serve every one. Do not care for service and gratitude in return. You are the Heir to the Infinite. All Power is behind you. But so long as you are a beggar, a beggar shall you remain. Renounce the lower self, Live for the Higher. What you call Universal Love is the expression on the lower plane of the subjective reception of ABSOLUTE UNITY on the Buddhic plane and in SAMADHI (Final Illumination).

LESSONS III AND IV.

THE YOGI SELF-DEVELOPER

INTRODUCTION.

In lessons 1 and 2 we have initiated you into the mysteries of Will and Mind-Force, the governing principles of the Universe and the laws of their development. We have also taught you how to acquire absolute control over Body and Mind. In these lessons we have striven to point out to you the right "Mental Attitude" towards your daily life, so that while mainly engaged in the task of Self-Culture you might also lend a hand in the great work of strengthening the race. Moreover our convictions, beliefs, and ideals are no mean, are insignificant factors in the determination of our health and environmental conditions. They react on our circumstances as well as on the WHOLE MAN. We have also given you important points of instruction in Soul Unfoldment, Meditation, Bramhacharya, Breathing, Fasting, Health-Culture, Body building and shown you, as distinctly as we could, the exact process of developing a single virtue in yourself thereby you may master the process and method of developing other virtues, the lines of action and thought being well-nigh similar in all, and focalizing at certain common points of primary importance. We have given the bare body of truth in connection with the development, evolution and unfoldment of the body and the soul, stripping of the metaphysical trappings and the theoretical draperies in which they are clothed. We have had to literally rend asunder the heavy wheel that had the divine face of truth. Hence our lessons are brief and to the point. We have had to contend against and overcome another serious difficulty. Expressed in the matter of fact English language, these wondrous truths of mysticism cannot but lose the air of profound solemnity and sanctity that pervades the subject of Yoga in Sanskrit literature. The wise and thoughtful student and we certainly do not write for light-headed and non-serious people, will not let their apparent simplicity deceive him or throw him off his guard. Rather let him realize that these lessons can be pressed into service in all directions and in all spheres of life. Let him just put them into practice and he will at once see their practical bearing on his daily life. These lessons do not go into the "WHAT" but point out the "HOW" of everything. We leave every student to suit his individual case as to the intellectual side of the ETERNAL PROBLEM. In conclusion we have to say that this Course does not pretend to deal with the advanced stages of Yoga, much less exhaust them. But they will, positively and decidedly prepare him for those higher things by lifting the PALL OF DARKNESS from his mind.

LESSONS III AND IV

Quite a number of you there must be to whom the "Fearless" mind is not only an enviable possession but something to which you are and have been an utter stranger. You may not say it to others—confession may hurt your pride—but secretly away deep in your heart, there resides strongly and fiercely the desire to be a Fearless Individual. And it is a worthy desire. To be able to wipe off all fearfulness, anxiety and worry from your mental tablets is no easy task, but when once accomplished, it gives you a glimpse of Heavenly Joy and Superhuman Strength. And, *You can be Fearless*, I tell you—each one of you—you can be what you will to be. I have seen it. I have done it. I am going to give you sound and positive instructions in this paper so that you may forge ahead towards your goal. These instructions are based upon good psychological grounds, have been tested and proved by millions and proved a blessing to whoever took them up in all earnestness and gave them a trial. If you want to be Fearless, hesitate not to follow them to the very letter.

I shall not waste space telling you about the dire results of fear, cowardice, worry, anxiety and the vile brood of negative thoughts branching of FEAR. Physically, mentally and spiritually man is what he thinks in his heart. As you think, so you are. Mind governs everything, creates or destroys everything, on the physical as well as other planes. Your thoughts affect your health, your circumstances, your environments; those who come into daily contact with you, those who are separated from you by space, those who are what you call "dead" but who are really alive in spirit-life and bound to you more or less by mystic chords of sympathy in thought and soul-life, affecting you and being affected by you every minute. The range of influence exerted by a man's daily thoughts is simply tremendous. Trees and animals, minerals and other objects of material life absorb it. The walls of your room, the clothes you wear, the letters you write are all being impressed by the aura of your thought-force. If you go to a clairvoyant or a psychometerist and put into his hands a letter, a lock of hair, a cloth-piece, or anything else pertaining to one of your friends, he or she will psychically trace out the personal appearance, temperament, past and present history, and everything else in connection with that person. Marvelous, 'Impossible' you cry in surprise. But it is done. Realize through study and investigation the importance of your thought-life and avoid vitiating it by fear-thoughts, hate-thoughts, sensual and sensuous thoughts and vanity thoughts. Because, mark you, these four giant-weeds poison the roots of the Tree of Life. All humanity suffers pain in diverse ways, on account of these four bad thoughts and their millions of off-springs. Now you will say this is all very well but:

HOW?

That is just what I mean to teach you all along. I don't want to feed you on mere empty theories, but I can and I will give you that knowledge which when assimilated shall build up strong flesh, bone, muscle, tissue, pith and marrow which will give you superb health, strength of mind and spirit—all of which are necessary adjuncts to Spiritual Growth and Happiness. Let me give you in detail methods and exercises. The ideal fearless man has many qualities. I say the Ideal Hero—no imitation patch work vulgarian. These qualities are in rough detail: (1) Devotion to God. (2) Knowledge. (3) Concentration. (4) Will Power. (5) Energy and Aspiration. (6) Health. (7) Self-Esteem. (8) Self-Control. (9) Love for Humanity. (10) Chastity. There may be other qualities but you will do well to build up the above and others will come to you by themselves. Let me drop a few helpful suggestions on the above. Follow each sentence closely.

1. DEVOTION TO THE ABSOLUTE WILL.

I have always said, written, observed and felt that the most courageous individuals are devoted to God. Such men are rare. You all understand the meaning of "Fearlessness" in its fullest sense. It means absolute independence—in two words, he is the FEARLESS man who "fears-nothing," and "faces-everything." That everything includes everyone. That nothing excludes no one. Viewed from this standpoint is not the fearless man rarely to be met with? You may come across degrees of fearlessness. Now the man who possesses this quality in the "highest degree" has faith in this God. Everyone has his conception of God. Everyone sees the absolute from his individual plane of vision. That conception which you have of God will do for you. I say, it will do for you and you alone. Don't force it upon others. Keep it for yourself. If you want to improve this conception of God pray in the Silence thus: "O, THOU, I UNDERSTAND NOT THY NATURE. I KNOW NOT—YET I YEARN TO KNOW. DO THOU REVEAL THYSELF UNTO MY SOUL. DO THOU OPEN MY SPIRITUAL EYES AND LEAD ME ON." Student, don't treat this lightly. Listen not to that conceited or blinded brother of yours who says he does not care for God—who says he can go on without the aid of God. Listen not. Listen not. The strongest and greatest pray often. Only they do not talk of this to others. They never make a show of their devotion. But they have all prayed and do all pray. They believe in personal effort—they also believe in Divine leading and guidance. Learn to be "lead by the Spirit." Everything shall come to you in this way. You will also notice that the Fearless Man is not a mere God-fearing man. He is a God-loving Individual. He loves God for God's sake largely. That man who is fearful in spite of his devotion to God is a sham devotee. But the grace of the LORD'S name is such that it shall purify the most impure of heart. It shall build up even a sham devotee into a real devotee who in time shall transcend all limitation. Therefore have faith in God. "Be regular" in your devotions. Also remember that each trial is a pain accompanying spiritual regeneration—each pain a process of strengthening the herald of a mere glorious dawn of wisdom. Hence give up a grumbling. The great God whose Infinite power regulates the motions of planets and yet takes note of the sparrow's fall has your soul's best interest at heart. All you do, all you say, all you feel, all you hope, all your experiences—all, all is His will. Man's Will is God's Will. God's Will is Man's Will. And who can define God? God alone has the power to define Himself. He has defined Himself as the Universe—Bramhanda. Nothing is impossible for the devotee of God. Let him but be willing to work and God shall give him everything. Regular devotion to God will surely develop extreme Fearlessness. "God is Love."

(2). KNOWLEDGE *(Gnayanam)*.

Fear is due to ignorance. When in the dark of night you mistook the rope for a snake, you shrieked out in terror. Cause? IGNORANCE. But when you saw the rope as a rope, you laughed out in amusement. Cause? KNOWLEDGE. All your fear is due to your ignorance of your real nature. All the fear at the last is fear of death. You have to realise through knowledge of the Vedanta that you are birthless, deathless. You have to unfold by meditation a consciousness of your Real Self. I give you hereunder a meditation exercise that will help you in this direction.

MEDITATION EXERCISE NO. 1.

Retire into the SILENCE. Shut off all thoughts and purposes relating to the external world. Try to realise that you, the Real Ego are not the body but that it is a mere garment you have put on for functioning on the physical plane and which you shall put off some day. Try to realise that you are immortal and that although a thousand bodies might come and go, you, the Ego, shall be as alive as ever. These are your shadows—your personalities. What dies and is born is a mirage— a mere phantasm—which you materialise for certain purposes. All these purposes centralise in one POTENTIALISED PURPOSE—the conquest of matter. Realise that you the Ego, have your dwelling in Supernal Regions—on the spiritual plane—with your Father-in-Heaven—but that you have come down into matter that you may find the fullest possible objective expression. Realise that you, the Ego, are a differentiated centre of consciousness in the Great Consciousness—THE ABSOLUTE—EGO—SUM of the entire Universe with all its gross and subtle manifestations—that you are endowed with all the powers and attributes of the Absolute Self. Realise that you are not the emotional and passional manifestations—surging up in your personality. These are subject to the law of Flux and Rhythm and must be brought under the control of Reason and Will—the balancing, equating principle of mind. Realize that you are not the mind nor the intellect, but that you exercise this function in order to analyze the external manifestations of nature and study same. Realize that you are pure Consciousness, Bliss and Existence in your essential nature—on with the all-life. Realize that the form side of manifestation is but a concentration, a precipitation within you. Your subjective nature is one with the subjective self of others—an inlet for the influx and efflux of the GREAT SUB-CONSCIOUS. Realize thus your Unity with All-Life-manifesting objectively as Universal Brotherhood of all living beings and the perfect recognition of the All-Father-Mother, the Great Cosmic Power and Intelligence known as God whose intelligence all-blissfulness and existence are ever pouring into each Unit of Individualized Divine Energy and evolving through nature. And, student, when you meditate daily that you are neither the body nor the emotions nor the mind, you shall then unfold the consciousness of the "I am I" that which rules the personality that which has been called Soul-Consciousness. You shall then be Chaitanya-Spiritually awake. You shall then know no Fear. Fear shall drop away like a worn-out sheath. All fear-thoughts are due to undeveloped race-consciousness which reacts upon individual consciousness and is stamped more or less upon every atom of matter. You 'fear' because you think you are the body. When you realize that you can command as many bodies for your use as you like; when you realize in your heart of hearts that you are a Spiritual Being expressing and energizing through material personalities; when you realize that you cannot die, fear shall be afraid of you and drop tormenting and teasing you. Fear resides in the matter-fed mind—that mind which has been grown and matured by the reception and re-action upon external sensations and stimuli—what has been called the objective mind. This mind identifies itself with the form, the body. It has an incorrigible determination towards the form-side, the concrete-side of existence. It sees nothing but the body and is darkened by the forces of *Maya*. It sees nothing but separation. Yes, it is the matter-fed mind. People with a development of this side of consciousness are invariably selfish; have generally small, conical eyes, understand nothing, but the welfare of the body. They are subject to the fear and the delight in making others fear them. This mind needs illumination from the soul, the Subjective Man, the "I am I" side of consciousness. It is not that you are a body and have a soul—this is the dirty conviction of the matter-fed mind—but you are a soul and have a body. The dawn of Soul-Consciousness makes a man a Force for good. He himself is Fearless. His is the voice of strength that does not crush and dominate but that puts warmth, life, energy, hope and indomitable courage into cold and despairing hearts. Some are born with this Soul-Consciousness. Do not think that I am feeding with the theories of eccentricity. Often when a boy playing with others the thought would strike me hard, "Are you the same that is running and jumping and shouting." I would stop, looking blankly ahead. A feeling of confusion would come over me and I would forget everything. I could recall the feeling distinctly and vividly. Now I understand. These were flashes of Soul-Consciousness unfolded in a past life and struggling for "recognition" in this life. Such men face DEATH for themselves calmly. They know they can't die. Such men are incapable of sustained hatred. They too have their physiognomical signs and distinctions. They represent an advanced order of intellect. And, lastly, when the full blaze of realization comes, your one object in life shall be to bestow your sense of freedom on others. You shall not be able to mock and smile calmly at the pain, the ignorance to imperfections of your brother-man. You shall realize what it is to 'feel' for humanity, yea, even for animals. You shall glimpse, in some measures, the great feeling of pain that rent the hearts of the Buddas, the Christs, the Ramakrishnas, the Vivekanandas of this world. They suffered, they felt for humanity. And when undeveloped humanity forced them to the Cross; they bore it in the same spirit in which the gentle nurse bears the blows and abuses of the disease-racked patient. "Father forgive them, for they know not what they do." Verily to know all is to forgive all. This Soul-Consciousness is as much yours as that of anyone. It comes through meditation on the Infinite, and the Formless Absolute—the Over-soul of the universe—the

Brahman of the Vedanta—the Self of the philosophers—the Atman of the Yogis—the personal—impersonal God of the devotee—and, last, but not least, the humanity of the humanitarian.

CONCENTRATION.

The mind can think of one thing only. Fear is an acute form of negative concentration—worry its chronic form. If you learn how to place your mind upon a particular subject and inhibit or "shut off" all other thoughts, the fascination of fear and worry shall have no power over you. Most of the things you fear never happen—others can be routed by a bold front. Even if something ugly does befall you, you have the power within to enable you to 'bear up' heroically. Fear is a mere negative thought-habit. It is a negative tendency in the mind. You can best eradicate this weed from your mind by cultivating the positive attitude of Courage. There are particular sets of brain-cells being created or destroyed by particular types of thoughts. The best way to destroy negative brain-cells is to develop positive brain-cells. If you want to *Kill off Fear-thoughts*, do not fight them. That would be like trying to realize how dark a place is and then starting to pitch it out by the handful. You know you cannot do it. Just open the blinds and let in sunshine and the place will be flooded with light. The mind hypnotized by negative thoughts has been compared by a mental scientist to a dirty wash-bowl full of dirty water. Take the wash-bowl near a tap and turn the tap on. The steady pour of clean water will soon wash off all the dirty water and fill the wash-bowl with clear water. So the only way to root out and destroy evil thoughts is to turn a steady stream of positive thoughts to overcome all fear thoughts, you should think courage-thoughts. Don't crawl on your belly; don't call upon Heaven to witness that despicable creature you are. No—a thousand times—no. Act Courage. Think Courage. Say Courage. That's the way. Turn your face towards the rising sun. Take "Courage" for your watchword. Affirm it as far as you can. Fasten it deep and strong in your mind. Always tell yourself that you are full of courage, morning, noon and night; never tell yourself that you are weak.

Now, in order to inhibit fear-thoughts and exhibit Courage-thoughts, you must possess CONCENTRATION. You should be able to take your mind off a certain subject and put it on something else at your will. Do you know what Concentration means? Let me give you in my own words something I remember reading about Napoleon. When banished to St. Helena and suffering from disease, one day his doctor expressed his curiosity as to the secret of his success and astonishing power. Napoleon replied "Doctor, there are drawers in my brain. When I want to think of politics I pull out the drawer of politics, when I want to think of Josephine, I pull out the drawer of Law, and so on; and when I shut all these drawers, I can go to sleep." The doctor smiled incredulity blandly. "Doctor, I can show you this minute. Doctor, I shut all drawers"—even while saying this, Napoleon fell with a thud on his pillow. He was fast asleep. The man of science and medicine examined him in all ways, but Napoleon had fallen actually fast asleep. This is Concentration and Mind-Control. I don't admire men of Napoleon's selfish types. Their place is in dark hell. They use their power for preying upon others. But that his powers of mind were great, I don't deny. Napoleon in his past life had been a great Yogi, but the remnants of self and cumulative force of bad Karma precipitated the bloody results you all know in connection with Napoleon's career. No doubt, this man was only a means used by God to bring about certain changes and revolutions.

To develop Concentration, pay attention to the daily work of your life. Don't neglect small things. Put interest and attention into whatever you think, say, or do. Be a wide-awake man. Don't go about your work half-asleep. Wake up and display a few signs of life. Be progressive. Think much and to the purpose.

WILL-POWER.

You all understand this. It is that aspect of your make-up that enables you to make your mind and body obey you. The true principle of Will is closely interlocked with the "I am I" as I have already explained it. Resolve at the start to do one thing once in 24 hours that you would do if you were not afraid. Face fear and it is your slave. Your Will-power enables you to prove things practically to yourself and to the world; to make actions match-thoughts. Give your Will much exercise in the right direction. Without Will a man is no better than a log of wood. Keep your Will strong by auto-suggestion and exercise. Try the powers of your Will on your personality till you can do anything and be anything. Say "I can and I will" in a thousand different ways and prove it too. The requisite qualities that form valuable adjuncts to Will-power are: 1. Determination. 2. Stick-to-it-ive-ness. 3. Perseverance. 4. Invincible and indomitable courage. 5. Non-attachment. 6. Faith in yourself. 7. Faith in God. 8. I can and I will. Repeat this affirmation often till it becomes a constant mental trait.

AFFIRMATIONS.

1. I am fearless. I am full of courage. There is nothing to fear. I say courage, I think, I act courage.

2. Courage is my distinct and leading trait. Everyone knows me as a man of Indomitable courage. The criticisms and opinions of others cannot affect me the least.

3. I am part of the Divine Self. I harm none. My nature knows no harm. Hence no harm comes to me.

4. I am equal to anything. Nothing can crush my spirit. I can face everything. I can face everybody.

5. My powers of resistance are strong, strong, strong. I use them never for the aggression of others. They are for my self-defense.

6. I am absolutely fearless morally and physically.

7. I stand for absolute truthfulness and justice and manifest them in myself.

8. Work with this affirmation. Strongly implant it in your mind. The use of strong, positive Affirmation in the Silence is valuable in that it gives you a firm hold of your thought so that you can "carry the thought" mentally. The value of expressing thought in act and speech lies in this that it clinches your thought into a permanent habit. Remember this psychological axiom: 1. Thoughts take form in action. 2. Action induces thought and corresponding habits. Therefore act out the part physically. If you want a courageous mind—"act out" the part physically, in your daily life, on suitable occasions, in all earnestness as you would in a theatre or drama. In a very short time it shall become a confirmed habit. Force yourself to it. Take an interest in what you do and say. Have confident expectations of SUCCESS. Never be daunted and cowed down by initial difficulties and failures. Never say die. If you go down—don't remain lying and moaning. Never, I say, never. Get up. Shake yourself up free and say, like the royal lion "Come one, come

all, this rock shall fly sooner from its base than I." Have a will of your own and be a force for good. Exercise your Will-power. Be something. Do something.

LOVE FOR HUMANITY, ENERGY, ASPIRATION, SELF-ESTEEM.

I cannot too strongly emphasize the difference between Self-Esteem and Self-Conceit. I wish to drive and thoroughly pound this difference into your brain. Self-Esteem is decidedly a manly trait. It is based upon a conviction of the Kingship of God and the Sonship of Man. Man is a dignified being with divine attributes. He should not disgrace his Maker by crawling on the ground. This is Self-Esteem. Self-Esteem does not lower itself. It never lowers others. You shall never see a leader of mankind without tremendous faith in himself. But equally truly you shall never see a true man or woman taking delight in having others crawl to dust before them. They feel pained and shocked at such a sight. There is infinite humiliation to them hi this sorry spectacle. But Self-Conceit is that original obliquity that leads a man to make a hog of himself. It is the old, dirty, unmanly "I-am-greater-than-you" feeling. Such men are hogs, hogs, hogs. They are not the true sons of their mothers. They are bastards and imbeciles. If you come across this type and get a chance to deal with him on your private strength open his eyes to his hoggishness. If he has any manly stuff in himself, he shall reform. If not, let him sizzle in his fat. Nature and its rigorous Laws will rub the lesson home someday. But don't you stand their nonsense for want of moral backbone. And the "I am" in you shall revolt against any such meanness and smallness in yourself. Encourage it not. Revere God. Revere yourself. Revere others. Next, as to energy and aspiration—these two characteristics transmute your mind from a negative into a positive type. They give you an aura of thought-force such as never knows fear. In point of fact fear is starved off to death. Be progressive. Take an interest in the affairs of this world and be a force for good. Raise yourself first. Then give others a lift. Have an Increasing Purpose in your life. Work towards its accomplishment. The man who renounces the world does not become a burden unto others. He helps others to shoulder their responsibilities. Nature aids at building up strong individuals. It has no use for barnacles and is always scraping them off. Nature does not tolerate leeches, vampires and parasites. Aspire to do something great in life "for the good of many, for the happiness of many." Live to some purpose. When you have a positive life-purpose, your tone of mind shall be dominant and positive and your thoughts shall match. All-strength shall come to you. Bad health, fear, worry and the whole array of disintegrating forces are set into active motion by a purposeless life. The Purposeful Man has no time to bother about them. Understand clearly, spirituality is not laziness, whatever else it may be.

AFFIRMATIONS.

1. I have perfect Self-Confidence. I am a Divine Being. I lower not myself—I lower not others.

2. My Life-Purpose is Constructive—not Destructive.

3. I will be great spiritually and mentally. I will make others great. I am an irresistible force for good.

4. I live to some great purpose. I am an Individual. I recognize the Fatherhood of God and the Brotherhood of man.

HEALTH, CHASTITY AND SELF-CONTROL.

Chastity and Self-Control bring to you a clean healthy physique. Strong health means strong brain. And strong brain means abounding vitality, magnetism and ambition. Remember our aim is the development of courage. The Chaste brain has tremendous energy. You should observe Bramhacharya—the conservation of vital energy in the body. You should acquire control over your passions and appetites. The energy generated in your body should not be drawn off at the lower end of your being, but should be transmuted into creative activity mentally and spiritually. Get a clean body, first. You can get it by fasting, breathing and exercise.

FASTING AND SELF-CONTROL.

If you feel heavy in body and brain, if you feel mentally sluggish it is a sure indication that your system is "clogged" with waste matter, due to partial or total inactivity of the physical channels of elimination. You have been indulging in high living and gluttony or you have been indulging in physical gratifications and have thus exhausted the vital fibers of your body. Perhaps you have drunk very little water which is nature's demand for cleaning the vessels of the body. Perhaps you have exercised little and thus the supply of oxygen required for burning off carbon and energizing the blood has been rather limited. Mental depression, 'weak nerves,' melancholy, despair, fear, lack of concentration and lots of other mental weakness are due to a clogging of the system with accumulated refuse. In brief, the following are a few of the benefits derivable from scientific fasting:—(1) It gives nature a chance to "Clean Up." The day of fasting is a day of physical "house cleaning." (2) Like the galvanic battery the body "recuperates" its energies. Strength is invariably rested to one's powers of digestion after a careful fast. No case of dyspepsia, constipation, etc., there is, but can benefit or be totally and radically cured by fasting. Fasting will increase powers of assimilation, quicken hunger, purify and strengthen the nerves and raise your health in all ways. (3) By gaining control over appetite you gain control over your lower nature. It is a splendid drill for your Will. You shall gain in spiritual strength. You shall grow positive to your flesh and its cravings. Jesus Christ fasted for 40 days in order to prepare himself to face his great trial and temptation. Our Yogis are all great fasters.

HOW TO FAST.

Don't undertake too much. If you have never observed a fast begin with a 24 hour fast. Drink at least 5, if possible, 8 tumblers of pure water at frequent intervals slowly. Keep yourself gently active and occupied the whole day, mentally and physically. You may feel a feeling of faintness, all-goneness and an irresistible craving for food. These are mischievous pranks of a cultivated and pampered and artificial appetite. Drink water slowly but don't give your body anything else. Always keep before yourself the distinction between the regal "I—am—I" the soul and the carnal, sensating animal known as the body. The great point of achievement during a fast lies in thinking high thoughts and forgetting the demands of the flesh. Don't think of your fast. If you do think say to yourself "this is to develop my will." Breathe plenty of fresh air. Exercise gently and walk. I have seen educated men afraid to go out for a walk during a day's religious fast "lest they should feel hungry." O shame! You can't control a little hunger! You should bathe daily thoroughly early in the morning, fast or no fast.

And don't be afraid. "Man liveth not by bread alone but by very word that proceeds from the mouth of God"—said Christ. Starvation may kill off your body but not fasting. Deny the power of all disease and weakness over yourself. Your mind is master of your body. Assert this mental control. Lastly, during a fast, your body is sensitive to your suggestions. Fill your mind with incessant affirmations of courage. Think courage, say courage, act courage. Take time by the forelock. Force your suggestions upon body and brain right now.

HOW TO BREAK A FAST.

When breaking a fast, be sure to control re-action. Eat very lightly and only sensible food. Now that you have a clean body, stay clean You can train yourself to fast for 40 days at a stretch.

TRANSMUTING SEX-ENERGY.

Here is some sensible advice from a leading thinker and teacher: To be a perfect Bramhacharin (a regenerate).

1. You must have a clean, healthy body; 2. Good breathing capacity and some control over same; 3. A strong will such as can move body and mind; 4. Assiduous cultivation of the intellectual side; 5. Control over emotions; 6. A fearless mind; 7. Great determination; 8. and abstemious living and high thinking.

The Yogis possess great knowledge regarding the use and abuse of the reproductive principle in both sexes. Some hints of this esoteric knowledge have filtered out and have been used by Western writers on the subject, and much good has been accomplished in this way. In this little book we cannot do more than touch upon the subject, and omitting all except a bare mention of theory, we will give a practical breathing exercise whereby the student will be enabled to transmute the re-productive energy into vitality for the entire system, instead of dissipating and wasting it in lustful indulgence in or out of the marriage relations. The re-productive energy is creative energy, and may be taken up by the system and transmuted into strength and vitality, thus serving the purpose of regeneration instead of generation. If the young men of the Western world understood these underlying principles they would be saved much misery and unhappiness in after years, and would be stronger mentally, morally and physically.

This transmutation of the reproductive energy gives more vitality to those practicing it. They will be filled with great vital force, which will radiate from them and will manifest in what has been called "personal magnetism." The energy thus transmuted may be turned into new channels and used to great advantage. Nature has condensed one of its most powerful manifestations of prana into productive energy, as its purpose is to create. The greatest amount of vital force is concentrated in the smallest area. The re-productive organism is the most powerful storage factory in animal life, and its force can be drawn upward and used, as well as expended in the ordinary functions of reproduction, or wasted in vicious lust. The majority of our students know something of the theories of regeneration, and we can do little more than to state the above facts, without attempting to prove them.

The Yogi exercise for transmuting re-productive energy is simple. It is coupled with rhythmic breathing, and can be easily performed. It may be practiced at any time, but is especially recommended when one feels the instinct more strongly, at which time the re-productive energy is manifesting and may be most easily transmuted for regenerative purpose. The exercise is as follows:—

Keep the mind fixed on the idea of energy, and away from ordinary sexual thoughts and imaginings. If these thoughts come into the mind do not be discouraged, but regard them as manifestations of a force which you intend using for the purpose of strengthening the body and mind. Lie passively or sit erect, and fix your mind on the idea of drawing the re-productive energy upward to the Solar Plexus, where it will be transmuted and stored away as a reserve force of vital energy. Then breathe rhythmically, forming the mental image of drawing up the re-productive energy with each inhalation. With each inhalation make a command of the Will that the energy be drawn upward from the reproductive organization to the Solar Plexus. If the rhythm is fairly established and the mental image is clear, you will be conscious of the upward passage of the energy, and will feel its stimulating effect. If you desire an increase in mental force, you may draw it up to the brain instead of to the Solar Plexus, by giving the mental command and holding the mental image of the transmission to the brain.

The man or woman doing mental creative work, or bodily creative work will be able to use this creative energy in their work by following the above exercise, drawing up the energy with the inhalation and sending it forth with the exhalation. In this last form of exercise only such portions as are needed in the work will pass into the work being done, the balance remaining stored up in the Solar Plexus.

You will understand, of course, that it is not the reproductive fluids which are drawn up and used, but the etheric prana energy which animates the latter, the soul of the reproductive organism, as it were. It is usual to allow the head to bend forward easily and naturally during the transmuting exercise.

Practise this Breathing Exercise sturdily. Be heroic. Learn to make 100 Pranayams at a sitting, but do not rush things. Deep breathing exercise, Will-Culture, regular Meditation and a clean normal mode of living when combined with much thinking will surely awaken your Latent Powers. Be not worried if progress be a bit slow at first. Keep up cheerful and work patiently. Things cannot but come your way if you don't give up but preserve to the last. Have infinite and unbounded faith in yourself. And, lastly, if you want to grow space in Wisdom and Power, persevere in deep breathing. Pranayam is the key to all spiritual success. "Spirituality is fullness of Breath." Almost all forms or Mental and physical weakness are due to imperfect and shallow breathing. Of all these instructions you practise nothing but the Breathing Exercise, your gain shall be great but in order to get all the results you must practise all the instructions regularly and methodically.

Your sex-force is under the direction of your sub-conscious mind which is quite amenable to your authoritative suggestions. Get control through your sub-consciousness. All you have to do is to let it to do its own work without adverse and negative suggestions and fear-thoughts. Say "No" vigorously to all adverse thoughts and shake them off from you. All health comes by letting nature alone.

BREATHING EXERCISE.

Find a quiet place as far as possible, where the air is pure and the surroundings soothing and pleasant. After a bath or a thorough rubbing of the body from top to toe, with a wet towel, on an empty stomach, take this exercise: Send a current of holy thought to everyone, on planes seen and unseen, north and south, east and west, engage in meditation—take anyone of the meditation exercises you like. When you are perfectly calm and relaxed, seat yourself cross-legged, assuming any posture that comes easiest to you, with head, neck and chest held in a straight line and the weight of the upper parts of the body resting on ribs. Keep the region about the waist quite free. Loosen the cloth there out and out. Now inhale air slowly and steadily through right nostril after closing left nostril with your finger as long as it takes to count sixteen mentally. Close both nostrils, holding the inspired air within and count sixty-four. Then very slowly exhale the air through the left nostril for as long as it takes to count thirty-two. You must begin with a 4 second inhalation, 16 second retention and 8 second exhalation. Instead of dry counting you might improve yourself decidedly by repeating the word "Fearless" as many times holding mentally that dominant idea back of the word. Practice 5 pranayamas mornings and evenings for one week daily. Increase to 10 next week. Work up to 20. Go slowly. Practice as long as you like, but not less than 6 months. Be serious and earnest. This is not for non-serious minds. This exercise will augment digestive power, steady heart-action, make the body light and the mind calm. It shall help also miraculously in your Soul-Unfoldment. During this practice be pure in all ways. Observe Bramhacharya. Practice mental concentration and spiritual meditation. Don't talk much with others. Don't encourage any but holy society. Don't sleep much. Don't work very hard. Keep your emotions well-in-hand. Be always engaged mentally and physically. Be hopeful and cheerful. Never encourage negative thinking. It shall do wonders for you.

PHYSICAL EXERCISE.

Exercise No. 1.

Stand straight, facing a corner of the room with bare feet about 14 or 15 inches from the corner itself, arms straight out, even with shoulders or perhaps two inches below, hands resting on the two-side walls, chest out, abdomen in. Now lean forward towards the corner, without moving the feet or bending the knees. Aim lightly to touch the corner with the chest, while holding the head and abdomen as far back from the corner as possible, arms and hands slipping forward on the walls in a straight line with shoulders. Resume first position without moving the feet or lowering the arms, and repeat. Make the forward movement slowly, at the same time inhaling through nostrils a slow, full breath; put your whole effort into stretching the chest forward and upward (careful not to bruise yourself against wall) and head and abdomen backward, thus straightening the back at the shoulders. Hold the chest to the corner a moment, holding the breath likewise, then slowly resume original upright position, slowly exhaling through slightly open lips at the same time bending the head forward towards the chest. As you lean forward toward the corner, mentally keep count of your exercise one, two, three, etc. As you resume the upright position, exhaling and bending the head forward mentally, affirm "I am fearless, pure, strong." Make these movements always slowly, deliberately, with the closest attention. Begin with 5 or 6 movements and raise to 20 at a time.

Exercise No. 2.

Stand straight about two feet from the wall. Place the palms on the wall-level with the shoulders. Without moving the feet or bending the body, lean forward slowly, inhaling slowly as you do so, until the chest touches the wall, head back; then push yourself slowly to an upright position slowly exhaling as you do so. Repeat 10 times or more.

Exercise No. 3.

Clasp the hands behind. As you slowly inhale extend the clasped hand slowly downwards as far as possible, straightening arms at elbow and lowering shoulders as much as possible, at the same time extending and lifting the chest as far as you can. Hold the breath and the position a moment only, shoulders down, chest out and up, abdomen in, then release the hand and slowly exhale. A rather vigorous exercise. So go slowly.

Exercise No. 4.

Stand straight, arms extended even with the shoulders, head up; tense muscles of right arm doubling slowly at elbow and hand only, until the clenched fist touches the shoulders; at the same time tensing the neck muscles, chin up, and turning the head slowly to face the clenched fist. Repeat with the left arm. The arms from shoulder to elbow must be kept in a horizontal position.

Exercise No. 5.

Stand straight, hands at sides. Bend as far over to the right as possible, slowly; then to the left as far as possible. Repeat 10 times.

Exercise No. 6.

Stand straight, arms at sides. Lean as far forward as you can without bending the knees and roll the body clear around in a circle to the right, arms and body as limp as possible. Repeat 5 times. Then roll five times to the left.

Exercise No. 7.

Stand straight. Extend arms easily in front. Wave them backwards and upwards in a sort of reversed swimming movement, until they meet overhead; at the same time bending backward as far as possible slowly inhale a full breath. Now bend forward, exhaling breath, taking care not to bend the knees, until your fingers touch your toes, head hanging as low as possible, toes and head as limp as possible, fingers reaching towards the floor. Repeat upright position. Keep the knees straight throughout. Aim to stretch the entire body and hands upward and backward as far as possible, with the upward motion of the arms. If you can't touch the floor without bending the knees, just come as near it as you can. Practice will limber you up until you can touch it.

Exercise No. 8.

Lie full length on the back of the floor, hands clasped under head. Tense the muscles of the right leg, raising the knee slowly until it touches or almost touches the body, at the same time bending the foot downward as far as possible, stretching the toes towards the floor. Now slowly lower the right leg, still tense, towards the floor, straightening the knee and turning the toe upward towards the body. As the right leg is being lowered, raise the left one upward in the same way tensing the muscles, knee to chest, toes stretching upward; as the left leg goes down, point the toes and foot toward the knee 5 times, increasing gradually to 10 times.

PHYSICAL EXERCISES.

SERIES 2.

Exercise I.

(1) Extend the arms straight out in front of you, on the level of the shoulder, with palms of the hand touching each other; (2) swing back the hands until the arms stand out straight, sideways, from the shoulders or even a little further back if they will go there easily without forcing; return briskly to position 1, and repeat several times. The arms should be swung with a rapid movement and with animation and life. Do not go to sleep over the work or rather play. This exercise is most useful in developing the chest, muscles of the shoulders, etc. In swinging the hands backward, it is an improvement if you will rise on your toe during the backward sweep; sinking on your heels as you move the arms forward again. The repeated movements should be rhythmical, backward and forward, like the swinging of a quick pendulum.

Exercise II.

(1) Extend the arms straight in front of you, letting the little fingers of each hand touch each other, the palms being upward; (2) then keeping the little fingers still touching, bring the hands straight up in a curved circular movement, until the tips of the fingers of both hands touch the top

of the head back of the forehead, the backs of the fingers touching, the elbows swinging out as the movement is made until (when the fingers touch the head, with thumbs pointing the rear) they point out straight sideways; (3) let the fingers rest on the top of the head a moment, and then with the elbows pressing back (which forces the shoulders back) force the arms backward with an oblique motion until they reach the sides at full length, as in the standing position.

Exercise III.

(1) Extend the arms straight out, sideways, from the shoulders; (2) then, still keeping the upper arms extended in same position, bend the arms at the elbow and bring the forearm upward with a circular movement, until the tips of the extended fingers lightly touch the tops of the shoulders; (3) then with fingers in the last position, force the elbows out to the front until they touch, or nearly go (a little practice will enable you to touch them together); (4) then, keeping the fingers still lightly touching the tops of the shoulders, swinging the elbows as far back as you can get them. (A little practice will enable you to get them much farther back than at the first attempt.) (S) Swing the elbows to the front position and then back to the rear position, several times.

Exercise IV.

(1) Place the hands on the hips, thumbs to the rear, and elbows pressed back; (2) bend the body forward, from the hips as far as you can, keeping the chest protruding and the shoulders pressed back; (3) raise the body to the original standing position (hands still at the hips) and then bend backward. In these movements the knees should not be bent and the motions should be made slowly and gently; (4) then (hands still on the hips) bend gently to the right, keeping the heels firmly on the ground, knees unbent and avoid twisting the body; (5) resume original position, and then bend the body gently to the left, observing the precautions given in the last movement. This exercise is somewhat fatiguing and you should be careful not to overdo it at the start. Proceed gradually; (6) with hands in same position on the hips, swing the upper part of the body around in a circle, from the waist-up, the head describing the largest circle, of course. Do not move the feet or bend the knees.

Exercise V.

(1) Standing erect, with hands on hips, raise yourself on the balls of the feet several times, with sort of a springing motion. Pause a moment after you have raised upon your toes, then let the heels sink to the floor, then repeat, as above suggested. Keep the knees unbent and the heels together. This exercise is especially beneficial in developing the calf of the leg, and will make it

sure the first few times it is tried. If you have an undeveloped calf here is the exercises for you; (2) with hands still on hips place your feet about two feet apart, and then cover the body into a "squatting" position, pausing a moment and then resuming original position. Repeat several times, but not too often at the first, as it will make the thighs feel a little sore at the beginning. This exercise will give one well developed thighs. This last movement may be improved upon by sinking down with the weight resting upon the balls of the foot, instead of upon the heel.

Exercise VI.

(1) Stand erect with hands on hips; (2) keeping the knee straight, swing the right leg out about fifteen inches (keeping the toe turned a little out and the sole flat)—then swing back to the rear until the toe points straight to the ground, *keeping the knee stiff all the time*; (3) repeat the swinging backward and forward several times; (4) then do the same with the left leg; (5) with hands still on hips, raise the right leg up, bending the knee, until the upper-leg (thigh) stands straight out from the body (if you can raise it still higher, you may do so); (6) place your foot again on the ground, and go through the same motion with the left leg; (7) repeat several times, first one leg and then the other, moving slowly at first and gradually increasing your speed until you are executing a slow trot without moving from the over spot.

Exercise VII.

(1) Stand erect, with the arms extended straight in front of you, from the shoulders, and of course on a level with the shoulders—the palms must be down, fingers straight out, thumbs folded under and the thumb side of hands touching each other; (2) bend the body forward from the hips, stooping forward as far as possible and at the same time swing the arms forward with a sweeping movement, sending them down, backward and upward at the back, so that when the body has reached the limit of the bending forward movement the arms are extended back and over the body—keep the arms stiff and do not bend the knees; (3) resume standing position and repeat several times.

Exercise VIII.

(1) Extend the arms straight, sideways, from the shoulder and hold them there stiff and rigid with hands open; (2) close the hands forcibly with a quick motion, pressing the fingers well into the palm; (3) open the hands forcibly and quickly, spreading out the fingers and thumbs as widely as possible forming a fan shaped hand; (4) close and open the hands as above stated, several times, as rapidly as possible. Put life into the exercise. This is a splendid exercise for developing the muscles of the hand and for acquiring manual dexterity.

Exercise IX.

(1) Lie upon your stomach, extending your arms above your head and then bowed upward and your legs stretched out full length and raised backward and upward. The correct position may be carried in the mind by imagining a watch—crystal or a saucer resting on the table on its middle, with both ends turning upward; (2) lower and raise the arms and legs, several times; (3) then turn over on your back and lie extended at full length, with arms extended straight out upwards over the head, with back of fingers touching the ground; (4) then raise up both legs from the waist until they stand straight up in the air, like the mast of a ship, your upper-body and arms remaining in the last position named. Lower the legs and raise them several times; (5) resume position 3, lying flat upon the back at full with arms extended straight out upward, over the head, with backs of fingers touching the ground; (6) then gradually raise body to sitting position, with arms projecting straight in front of the shoulders. Then go back gradually to the lying down position, and repeat the raising and lowering several times; (7) then turn over on the face and stomach again and assume the following position:—Keeping the body rigid from head to foot, raise your body until its weight rests upon your palms (the arms being stretched out straight in front of you) at one end, and upon your toes at the other end. Then gradually bend arms at the elbow, allowing your chest to sink to the floor; then raise up your chest and upper-

body by straightening out your arms, the entire weight falling upon the arms, with the toes as a pivot—this last is a difficult motion, and should not be overdone at first.

Exercise X.

This exercise is for those troubled with a too large abdomen, which trouble is caused by too much fat gathering there. The abdomen may be materially reduced by a reasonable indulgence in this exercise—but always remember "moderation in all things" and do not overdo matters, or be in too much of a hurry. Here is the exercise: (1) exhale the breath (breathe out all the air in the lungs, without straining yourself too much) and then draw the abdomen in and up as far as you can, then hold for a moment and let it resume its natural position. Repeat a number of times and then take a breath or two and rest a moment. Repeat several times, moving it in and out. It is surprising how much control one may gain over these stubborn muscles with a little practice. This exercise will not only reduce the fatty layers over the abdomen, but will also greatly strengthen the stomach muscles. (2) Give the abdomen a good but not rough kneading and rubbing.

Exercise XI.

The exercise is as follows:—Follow it carefully. (1) stand erect, with heels together, toes slightly pointed outward; (2) raise the arms up by the sides (with a circular movement) until the hands meet over the head, thumbs touching each other; (3) keeping the knees stiff; the body rigid; *the elbows unbent*; (and shoulders bent well back as the movement is made); bring down the hands, slowly, with a sideway circular motion, until they reach the sides of the legs the little finger and the inner-edge (the "chopping-edge") of the hand alone touching the legs, and palms of the hands facing straight to the front. The shoulder gets the right position by touching the little finger of each hand to the seam of the trousers. (4) Repeat several times, *slowly* remember. With the hands in the last position, having been placed there by the motion stated, it is very difficult for the shoulders to warp forward. The chest is projected a little; the head is erect; neck is straight, the back straight and hollowed a little (the natural position); and the knees are straight. In short, you have a fine, erect carriage—*now keep it*.

SEVEN MINOR BREATHING EXERCISES.

Exercise I.

(1) Stand erect with hands at sides. (2) Inhale complete breath. (3) Raise the arms slowly, keeping them rigid until the hands touch overhead. (4) Retain the breath a few minutes with hands over head. (5) Lower hands slowly to sides exhaling slowly at the same time. (6) Practice cleansing breath.

Exercise II.

(1) Stand erect with arms straight in front of you. (2) Inhale complete breath and retain. (3) Swing arms back as far as they will go; then back to first position; then repeat several times, retaining the breath all the while. (4) Exhale vigorously through mouth. (5) Practice cleansing breath.

Exercise III.

(1) Stand erect with arms straight in front of you. (2) Inhale complete breath. (3) Swing arms around in a circle, backward, a few times. Then reverse a few times retaining the breath all the while. You may vary this by rotating them alternately like the sails of a wind-mill. (4) Exhale the breath vigorously through the mouth. (5) Practice cleansing breath.

Exercise IV.

(1) Lie on the floor with your face downward, and palms of hands flat upon the floor by your sides. (2) Inhale complete breath and retain. (3) Stiffen the body and raise yourself up by the strength of your arms until you rest on your hands and toes. (4) Then lower yourself to original position. Repeat several times. (5) Exhale vigorously through the mouth. (6) Practice cleansing breath.

Exercise V.

(1) Stand erect with your palms against the wall. (2) Inhale complete breath and retain. (3) Lower the chest to the wall, resting your weight on your hands. (4) Then raise yourself back with the arm muscles alone, keeping the body stiff. (5) Exhale vigorously through the mouth. (6) Practice cleansing breath.

Exercise VI.

(1) Stand erect with arms "akimbo" that is with hands resting around the waist and elbows standing out. (2) Inhale complete breath and retain. (3) Keep legs and hips stiff and bend well forward, as if bowing, at the same time exhaling slowly. (4) Return to first position and then take another complete breath. (5) Then bend backward exhaling slowly. (6) Return to first position and take a complete breath. (7) Then bend sideways exhaling slowly (vary by bending

to right and then to left). (8) Practice cleansing breath.

Exercise VII.

(1) Stand erect or sit erect with straight spinal column. (2) Inhale a complete breath but instead of inhaling on a continuous steady stream, take a series of short, quick "sniffs" as if you were smelling aromatic salts and ammonia and did not wish to get too strong a "whiff." Do not exhale any of these little breaths, but add one to the other until the entire lung space is filled. (3) Retain for a few seconds. (4) Exhale through the nostrils in a long restful breath. (5) Practice cleansing breath.

WHEN YOU ARE IN TRAINING.

Do not attempt to take all the above exercises at one and the same time. Take them several times in the day. Never exercise immediately after a meal or before it. Do not try to force development as you will be apt to suffer from re-action. Slow and steady wins the race. Gentle and persistent exercises are advisable. That will lead to permanent development.

EFFECT OF MIND AND BODY.

It has been proved conclusively even on the physical plane that a "a Man thinks in his heart so is he." The great thing to avoid is Fear and Worry thoughts. These and all other undesirable thoughts are due to bad health partially but it is even a greater truth that physical degeneration is due to bad thinking. Fear affects the heart. During epidemics such as plague, cholera, etc., you generally first project the deadly germs of Fear-Thoughts upon yourself and thus by weakening your mind you weaken your body and expose yourself to disease influence. Again, if you have some hereditary disease and if you accept adverse suggestions from ignorant people and keep telling yourself that such and such a disease has taken shelter in you and your body as its "fixed abode" you simply hasten your own end. The body and mind are interrelated. Thoughts materialize themselves in your body. You should get as far away from the idea of disease and old age and weaknesses as possible and hold the health-thoughts steadily before your mind. The only way in which to be quite immune from Disease is to Deny the Power of Disease on yourself. Say "I cannot be ill," "I will not admit disease." Health and strength are in the unyielding will. De-hypnotize yourself of that superstition that God sends disease. Your body is yours to control and keep healthy. God will give you—(He has already given you rather)—the Power to control your body. Remember always; you alone can save yourself. All Power and

Wisdom are potentially resident in you. Have confidence and set that thing in motion, exercise it constantly and persistently and it shall grow and unfold. God is in you and you are in God. When you pray you are simply, although often unconsciously, helping that Latent Power to uncoil itself. Remember again: God will grant you the opportunity, the means, the wisdom, the ability to accomplish a thing, but You Shall Have to do the work yourself. Hence, you see, the illumined mind is quite necessary for perfect health. Get rid of all weak thoughts. Have a strong mind. Remember lastly:

MIND ACTS UPON BODY IN ALL WAYS.

Make your mind positive to your body. I have told you how to do so. Physical exercise plus Mental Exercise will put you on the road to Power and Poise. And side by side with this follow health-laws. But bear in mind that if you assert your power on your mind and body confidentially, they cannot but obey your commands. The body has an intelligence of its own. This intelligence knows its work perfectly. It is what you call Instinct. It digests your meals; assimilates and eliminates; repairs wastes; works the heart and controls the circulation; heals wounds and presides over all other natural and involuntary processes in the body. This Instinctive mind knows its work perfectly. But, mark you, this intelligence in the cells and nerve-centers of your body is negative to the Central

Intelligence in the brain—the controlling center—the "I Am" and is affected by suggestions, beliefs and thoughts in your brain. All you have got to do is to avoid projecting negative thoughts from your mind and let it alone. But suppose you have by violation of the Laws of Nature disturbed the action of the Instinctive Mind, disease results. Disease is simply the effect of nature to throw off unnatural conditions and re-assert natural conditions. In such a case all you have got to do is to re-establish natural states. You can do so by simply increasing the general vitality of the body and by changing your Mental Attitude. For instance, if you somehow or other have accepted the "belief" that your stomach is weak or your heart is weak or your liver is slow or your circulation is bad or your vitality is low, etc., your instinctive Mind will take up your Beliefs and work them out in no time physically. The Instinctive Mind—which is the same as the sub-conscious Mind working in the body—*never reasons*. It is on the plane of Automatism. Therefore, if you have done any such negative thinking your first step is to wipe out these noxious mental weeds by the Positive Denial. Say "No, No, No, my body is strong; my stomach is strong, my heart is strong, etc." In this form of suggestion you use positive Denial as well as Positive Affirmation. The former is destructive of evil if rightly applied; the latter is constructive of good. Belief and confident expectation are mighty forces. Be sure you apply them wisely. The power of mind over matter is supreme and a Proven Reality.

RESERVE FORCE.

Here I should like to draw your attention to the Reserve Power existing in your body. Of course there are soul-powers existing potentially within YOU which leap into brilliant expression as you succeed in developing and expanding your brain to a state of perfect responsiveness to the touch of your will. For really and truly your will, forming as it does the divine part of yourself, is always strong and must unfold "as a rose" by exercising itself, in the field of matter, force and mind;—all of which are subordinate to YOU and the real aim of human evolution is actually to place in your hands the wand of power.

What is within your body is sure to find its correspondent outside in Nature. Control nature inside and you will move as a master out in this universe.

Now without going into details let me tell you—if you do not know it already—that mind is the finest form of matter, and matter the grossest form of mind, and there is a constant interaction between the two poles. But since mind represents the positive end and matter the negative, the former can dominate the latter. You can evoke states of consciousness by applying stimulus to the periphery and again mental states evoke corresponding vibrations in the cellular life of body and brain.

Hence you see your mind controls and forms your body. Also your body reacts upon your brain and affects that part of your mind which has to operate through the brain, which is matter pure and simple. So to keep aright the polarities of your brain and body a constant adjustment of forces is needed and thus you can establish POISE.

In order always to be in a state of perfect health two things are necessary. Deny the power of disease over yourself. In the unyielding will is health. In the weak, vacillating, fearful mind is disease and death. At the same time always be in perfect magnetic trim with the physical laws of health. A knowledge of the latter and the ascension of a fearless mental attitude will open up hitherto unrecognized channels of physical and mental expression. Physiological researches have led sincere investigators to the inevitable conclusion that there is subtle, refined, dynamic substance, a reality that binds up the reorganization, causes growth, vitality and motion; repairs injuries; makes up losses; overcomes and cures diseases. Von Helment called it "Archeus"; Stahl called it "Anima;" Whytt called it the "sentiment principle;" Dr. Cullen called it "Caloric;" Dr. Darwin called it "Sensorial energy"; Rush called it "Occult cause;" and many other names such as "Vital Principle," "Living power," "Conservative Power," "Odic

Force," etc., etc., have been given to it. We of India have recognised it and devised Yoga methods for controlling it; we call it Prana and only in India do you come across men who possess pranic control or control over universal energy.

There exists in your physical organism reserve stores of vital energy stored away for your use, particularly in that central ganglion of your vital battery known as the Solar Plexus and generally in the chain of ganglia or storage batteries along and up your spine and elsewhere in other nerve-centers. The solar plexus is also known as the Abdominal Brain and your brain depends and draws upon this vital centre for its energies. You will find after the prolonged concentration and brain-work that this part of your body—at the back of pit of stomach—becomes warm. Now when you engage in physical exercise, for instance, you must have noticed how at first you soon get tired and all done up. But if you wait a little and then start again, you will find how the sense of fatigue has quite passed away and you can run your body under full pressure for a very long time, and the more you exert yourself the greater and more powerful the surging up of your vital energy. With each new exertion you seem to acquire a fresh start. This has puzzled physiologists. You will find a parallel phenomenon in mental work. You may experience a sense of weariness and fatigue in some brain-work which demands close thinking and attention, but if you attack your work a little later after the first effort you will do your work a surprising degree of freshness, vigour, and enthusiasm far surpassing the original attempt. Again everyone can and does put forth universal energy under pressure of some urgent necessity, which will startle even himself. No matter who you are and what your physical condition, there is an enormous amount of power in your body that has never been drawn upon at all and impatiently waiting for up-call. We go on in ordinary dog trot pace, resting, limping, "taking care of our health," and then we think we are doing our best. Do not permit your mind to be self-hypnotized into a false sense of being "exhausted" and "old." Neither of them is a fact except in your thought of yourself. All your powers are lying dormant. All your latent energies are lying unused. Back of your conscious mentality are tremendous energies awaiting the pull of your will. When your brain conceives of being something unusually great, at least so it may appear from your view-point, do not question your strength but go ahead unhesitatingly, fearlessly and steadily. Assert your life-force. Feel that you are young, strong and healthy and fit. Live in mental consciousness of power and never think of weakness. Keep your grip and run right along. Nature is sure to honor your draft. Nature is sure to give you strength, energy and vim, in boundless measure. Just try this my friends, you, who write me of "there being a serious lack of vitality" in your system and hence your inability to grapple with the occult. No such thing. Fact is you lack courage and initiative, pluck and "go" and you are laboring under the hypnotism of weakening thoughts. Just change your thoughts, and your reserve forces will rush out into activity and you will be a changed man in no time.

HOW TO EXERCISE.

In exercising aim at rhythm of motion. Let your movements be easy, regular, rhythmic and graceful. Take an interest in your work. Do pay attention. Put Will-Power and Mind into your work. Think of all it means. Do not fatigue yourself unduly. After exercise towelling or a spray-bath is advisable. Wet your towel, pass it over your body, rubbing thoroughly. Raise the towel and repeat. After exercise and towelling, you should be in a splendid glow. Be sure to keep the windows open when exercising. Fresh air is an absolute necessity. Never mind about cold and so forth. Remember the Positive Denial will fill you with Power of Resistance. Say "Cold cannot affect my body" and believe what you say. You can face anything in this way and remain untouched.

BATHING AND LINEN.

The student should bathe daily, using plenty of water, rubbing and cleaning the body from top to toe. I myself bathe very early in the morning, in all seasons, in cold water. Cold water stimulates circulation and is a wonderful tonic internally and externally. Warm water is soothing and relaxing in its effect. If you can bathe in the flowing water of a river, so much the better. Swimming is a wonderful bracer, besides being an enjoyment in itself. There is Prana in water and your body extracts this Prana from air, water and food. I cannot give you instructions as to different forms of bathing, as this is not a "doctor" book. As far as possible bathe twice a day, mornings and evenings; if not, once in the morning, using the towel at other times. Bathing is not merely pouring water on body but cleansing it out and out with water rubbing and scrubbing with hands and towels. Aim at perfect cleanliness. Cleanliness is Godliness and Health is Holiness.

Then again while bathing if you let the water flow over your body and try to "appreciate the sensation" and dwell on the idea of Prana-absorption from water, you shall get double benefit.

About linen—*Be neat*, for God's sake. I have seen orthodox people who bathe twice and wash their hands hundreds of times in the day, but whose clothes are sticky with dirt, sweat and oil.

Whatever else it may mean, Religion does not mean squalor, offensive odors in body and clothes and general neglect of external clean linen and dirt. The Yogi is a man of supreme REFINEMENT. Read that word and understand all it means. The clothes you wear in day-time should not be worn at night. Be clean internally as well externally. Be clean. Be clean. Be clean, within as well as without.

DRINKING WATER
AND SWALLOWING AIR.

Your body needs a reasonable supply of water and air. Water is used by nature in different ways. Form the habit of drinking pure water from 5 to 8 tumblers a day. Drink slowly and form a mental image of Prana-absorption from the water.

The student needs fresh air too in plenty. If your heart and lungs are in sound condition they will draw in air naturally and extract oxygen in proper quantities. If not, perform the following exercises carefully one by one in the open air every day. They are quite reliable.

THE YOGI CLEANSING BREATH.

(1) Inhale a complete breath. (2) Retain the air a few seconds. (3) Pucker up the lips as if for a whistle (but do not swell out the cheeks) then exhale a little air through the opening with considerable vigor. Then stop for a moment retaining the air and then exhale a little more air. Repeat until the air is completely exhaled. Remember that considerable vigor is to be used in exhaling air through the opening in the lips. This breath will be found quite refreshing when one is tired and generally "used up." A trial will convince the student of its merits. This exercise should be practiced until it can be performed naturally and easily, as it is used to finish up a number of other exercises given in this book and it should be thoroughly understood.

NERVE VITALISING BREATH.

(1) Stand erect. (2) Inhale a complete breath and retain same. (3) Extend the arms straight in front of you, letting them somewhat limp and relaxed, with only sufficient nerve force to hold them out. (4) Slowly draw the hands back towards the shoulders gradually, contracting the muscles and putting force into them, so that when they reach the shoulders the fists will be so tightly clenched that a tremulous motion is felt. (5) Then keeping the muscles tense push the fists slowly out and then draw them back rapidly (still tense) several times. (6) Exhale vigorously through the mouth. (7) Practice the cleansing breath. (8) The efficiency of this exercise depends greatly upon the speed of the drawing back of the fists, and the tension of the muscles, and, of course upon the full lungs. This exercise must be tried to be appreciated. It is without equal as a "bracer" as our western friends put it.

THE VOCAL BREATH.

(1) Inhale a complete breath very slowly, but steadily, through the nostrils, taking as much time as possible in the inhalation. (2) Retain for a few seconds. (3) Expel the air vigorously in one great breath, through the wide-opened mouth. (4) Rest the lungs by the cleansing breath. This would give you a good, rolling voice.

THE RETAINED BREATH.

(1) Stand erect. (2) Inhale a complete breath. (3) Retain the breath as long as you can comfortably. (4) Exhale vigorously through the open mouth. (5) Practice the cleansing breath. At first you will be able to retain the breath only a short time, but a little practice will also show a great improvement. Time yourself with a watch, if you wish to note your progress.

CELL STIMULATION.

(1) Stand erect with hands in sides. (2) Breathe in very slowly and gradually. (3) While inhaling, gently tap the chest with the fingertips, constantly changing position. (4) When the lungs are filled, retain the breath and the chest with the palms of the hands. (5) Practice the cleansing breath.

RIB STRETCHING.

(1) Stand erect. (2) Place the hands one on each side of the body as high up in the armpits as convenient, the thumbs reaching towards the back, the palms on the side of the chest and the fingers to the front over the breast. (3) Inhale a complete breath. (4) Retain the air for a short time. (5) Then gently squeeze the sides at the same time slowly exhaling. (6) Practice the cleansing breath.

CHEST EXPANSION

(1) Stand erect. (2) Inhale a complete breath. (3) Retain the air. (4) Extend both arms forward and bring the two clenched fists together on a level with the shoulder. (5) Then swing back the fists vigorously until the arms stand out straight sideways from the shoulders. (6) Then bring back to position (4) and swing to position (5). Repeat several times. (7) Exhale vigorously through the open mouth. (8) Practice the cleansing breath.

WALKING EXERCISE.

(1) Walk with head up, chin drawn slightly in, shoulders back, and with measured tread. (2) Inhale a complete breath, counting (mentally) 1, 2, 3, 4, 5, 6, 7, 8, one count to each step making the inhalation extend over the eight counts. (3) Exhale slowly through the nostrils, counting as before 1, 2, 3, 4, 5, 6, 7, 8, one count to a step. (4) Rest between breaths, continuing, walking and counting 1, 2, 3, 4, 5, 6, 7, 8, one count to a step. (5) Repeat until you begin to feel tired. Then rest for a while and resume at pleasure. Repeat several times a day. You may vary the exercise by retaining the breath during a 1, 2, 3, 4, count and then exhale in an eight-step count. Practise whichever plan seems most agreeable to you.

MORNING EXERCISE.

(1) Stand erect in a military attitude, head up, eyes front, shoulders back, knees stiff, hands at sides. (2) Raise body slowly on toes, inhaling a complete breath, steadily and slowly. (3) Retain the breath for a few seconds, maintaining the same position. (4) Slowly sink the first position at the same time slowly exhaling the air through the nostrils. (5) Practice cleansing breath. (6) Repeat several times, varying by using right leg alone, then left leg alone.

STIMULATING CIRCULATION.

(1) Stand erect. (2) Inhale a complete breath and retain. (3) Bend forward slightly and grasp a stick or cane steadily and firmly, and gradually exerting your entire strength upon the grasp. (4) Relax the grasp, return to first position, and slowly exhale. (5) Repeat several times. (6) Finish with the cleansing breath. (N. B.—*The above are from the Yoga Teachings.*)

MEDITATION EXERCISE No. I.

Retire into the silence. Say: I AM FEARLESS. Concentrate calmly on that idea. Think it out in all its bearings. See yourself in your mind's eye as possessing the desired quality and acting it out in actual life. Let your mind indulge in a good, strongly-dramatized day-dream. Only insist upon its sticking to the particular text of thought and always showing you successful at the end. Finish up with a vigorous affirmation of the "I am." Practise at the same hour daily for 6 months at least.

Exercise No. II.

Retire into the silence. Concentrate earnestly thus: *I send out strong, positive, healing thought-waves of love to all mankind. Let the disease-ridden become healthy. Let the weak become strong. Let the needy ones become prosperous and happy. Let the fearful ones become filled with courage. Let the cruel become kind and merciful. Let the hateful and hating ones become loving. Let the impure ones become pure. Let the bereaved, deserted, sorrow-stricken ones become soothed and comforted.*

Picture to yourself strong waves of Thought-Force passing out of you and encircling the whole world. Picture the world as peopled with men and women manifesting the desired conditions.

The more friends sit together in union of will and soul concentrating as above-indicated the better. Practise alone if you can find no earnest and serious-minded ones to join you.

Believe in your power to so help humanity. The power of thought is unlimited. In blessing others bless yourself. The effect of this exercise will be far-reaching. It shall follow and be a blessing to you even after death. Practise regularly at the same place and time as far as possible.

Be earnest in your work.

Do not talk of your exercises to others.

The above exercises will wonderfully develop and strengthen anyone who tries them. The deep breathing exercise already given is known as Pranayama or Controlling the Psychic Breath. Its main purpose is to give you control over your Prana and unfold the Psychic Force latent in you. Practised on an impure body and weak lungs it may do harm. Hence students are advised to undergo the above 10 breathing exercises first and then, when their lungs have developed the power of endurance, they should take that up. It will take time, patience, and serious work. But if the student is sufficiently energetic he will perfect all these exercises in six months. But follow nature's plan and be slow and steady.

DIET.

You all know that pure food brings pure blood. You should avoid the two extremes of gluttony and daily fasting and abstemiousness. You should know (1) What to eat (2) How to eat (3) When to eat.

Concentrated food such as contains the maximum amount of nourishment in a minimum quantity should be used. The student should study some reliable hand book on the relative values of food and use his judgment. We ourselves use nuts, milk, fruits, whole wheat bread, rice in very small quantity, pulse, etc. Those who are non-meat eaters—and we advise it strongly—will do well to see to it that their *menu* has a good supply of albuminous food, as vegetarians often run the risk of being overfed as to starch and underfed in nitrogenous foods.

(2) Chew and masticate properly so as to extract the food-Prana in full and break up the food-substance into very small bits, reducing it to pulp. Do not be in a hurry to bolt your food but let it linger in your mouth so as to be properly insalivated and so that the nerves of the tongue, cheek, etc., may all absorb energy from food. Remember your stomach is not lined with rows of teeth. This will give you double the nourishment you get ordinarily, avoid constipation, prevent malnutrition, non-assimilation and over-eating. Out of a very small

quantity of food you can extract perfect nourishment and thus you avoid loading and "stuffing" the stomach with unnecessary food. It is also economical in case you are a thrifty soul! Eat to live. Don't live to eat.

(3) Eat when you are hungry. That cultivated "appetite" that craves for satisfaction at certain stated intervals of the day and brings on an "all-gone" fainting, nauseating sensation in the stomach is not real "hunger." In real hunger there is absolutely no sensation in the stomach but there is a rich and continuous flow of saliva in the mouth and that sort of thing makes you enjoy the plainest of fares. Even a dry crust of bread will taste sweet as Manna. Cut off your breakfasts. Drink cold water instead. Eat one good, nourishing meal at 12 A. M., and one light meal in the evening.

Lastly, students, let plain living and high thinking be your motto. Do not be afraid to eat when you are hungry and so long as you exercise and work with brain and body even two square meals a day are permissible. Do not grow ethereal and airy, because then you will not amount to much in the world's work. Students, who are perfect Brahmacharies, will not care half as much for lots of food as ordinary folk do. A constant feeling of satisfaction and fullness is present in such. But hard workers must never present in such. But hard workers must never be under-nourished and they require more food than others.

SLEEP.

It is the depth and relaxation in sleep that counts. High-strung people find it hard to relax and keep tossing on their pillows. Bathe your feet in cold water in hot season and in cool water in cold season. That will draw off the surplus blood gurgitating in your brain. Also bathe the nape of the neck. The student should engage in meditation before falling to sleep, as during sleep the Man leaves the physical form and goes to super-physical planes and it is the last train of thought in your mind that determines and conforms you to the special super-physical influence you are to obtain. The physical benefits too shall be great. You will feel more rested in this way and your sleep will be sleeping a sounder and more refreshing sleep than otherwise. One of the chief signs of success in Mental and Physical Control is that your sleeps are undisturbed and peaceful.

During sleep you are in a passive, relaxed condition and all sorts of unseen influences play around you. It is good therefore to enclose yourself in an Astral Shell. Concentrate upon your aura and picture it as extending some 18 inches all around you and forming a shell around you. Now take this affirmation to concentrate your mind.

1. I am charging my aura with my Will-Force.

2. It is strong, strong, strong and can and will resist, repel and drive off all bad influences and admit only pure and holy influence.

3. It will remain around me right along the period of my sleep.

The student is advised to surround himself in this "auric Shell" even when awake so that it may beat off all malign and harmful thought-forces. As he grows in Will-Power and Self-Confidence, a Protective Aura will form around him naturally and will be felt by others.

RELAXATION VERSUS CONTRACTION.

The student should learn to relax his body completely so that it shall lie still and limp and soft as cotton. He should be able to tense and contract his muscles so that they will become hard as iron. In all the physical exercises you will find two special actions (1) Muscle contraction (2) Stretching. When you contract muscle and harden it, you have sent currents of nerve-force and will to that part; when you relax it, you "let go" completely. What we want is Strength in Repose ready to leap into action in the flash of an eye. We have taught you how to relax in Lesson 2 on Will-Force. You all have noticed a cat crouching for its prey. How intensely still it is; yet you know what such stillness means. It is very far from laziness. Relaxation husbands and conserves nerve-force. It is a great thing to be calm and silent. Calmness is the centralization of tremendous power. Practice being calm, as far as you can.

SOLAR ENERGY.

There is great electrical and thermal power in the sun's rays. If the human body be properly exposed to the sun during the first five hours in the morning and the evening, the body would absorb energy therefrom and gain in strength. Do not over do this, especially you of the warm climate.

LAST WORD ON HEALTH.

Trust Nature. It is her office to keep your body-machine running in perfect order. "Prevention is better than cure"—they say. Observe the healthy man. See how he lives and follow his example. But note that body is yours to control and God will not do that work for you. Also get rid of the stupidity that God sends diseases. Think, study and observe and you will know what Health Laws are.

CONCLUSION

Student, I have indicated the lines along which you are to seek the way to Spiritual Independence. I cannot run your life-affairs, solve your life-problems, do your work for you. I have pointed out a few principles, observe, think and complete your knowledge. You must climb the steps of the ladder of attainment and Self-Perfection yourself.

Fear is a great stumbling-block in the way. Fight it down. Starve it out. Be earnest. Be thorough. Live your life silently and earnestly. Give others a helping hand whenever you can without that patronizing air of superiority so characteristic of the modern snobs passing for "gentlemen." Be proud that you are an "Indian." Follow Indian ideals of greatness. Consider it a privilege to help deserving souls. We all need help, encouragement and guidance to some extent. Co-operation, interdependence are the basic foundations of human well-being. Be strong. Be manly. Be courageous. Be great and good. Take your place in the world's evolutionary progress and lend your hand in turning the wheel of life. In the same measure that you help others, shall you yourself be helped on all planes of life. Be reasonable. Be just and fair unto others. Be a source of blessing unto others. So long as you labor under the vitiating influence of negative thoughts, you cannot achieve much in any direction. I have told you "how" you are to proceed.

May God bless you. May he guide, help and strengthen where I have failed.

SWAMI MUKERJI.